Self Assessment in Clinical Pharmacology

D R Laurence MD FRCP
Professor Emeritus of Pharmacology and Therapeutics,
School of Medicine, University College London, London, UK

P N Bennett MD FRCP
Consultant Physician, Royal United Hospital, Bath and Reader in Clinical
Pharmacology, University of Bath, Bath, UK

M J Brown MSc MD FRCP
Professor of Clinical Pharmacology, University of Cambridge; Consultant
Physician, Addenbrooke's Hospital, Cambridge and Director of Studies
Gonville and Caius College, Cambridge, UK

THIRD EDITION

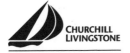
CHURCHILL
LIVINGSTONE

EDINBURGH LONDON NEW YORK PHILADELPHIA SYDNEY TORONTO 1999

CHURCHILL LIVINGSTONE
An imprint of Harcourt Brace and Company Limited

© D. R. Laurence, P. N. Bennett, M. J. Brown 1999

🏋 is a registered trade mark of Harcourt Brace and
Company Limited

Originally published as MCQs in Clinical Pharmacology
First published 1983
Second edition 1988
Third edition 1999

ISBN 0 443 06125 4

British Library Cataloguing in Publication Data
A catalogue record for this book is available from the
British Library.

Library of Congress Cataloging in Publication Data
A catalog record for this book is available from the
Library of Congress.

Medical knowledge is constantly changing. As new
information becomes available, changes in treatment,
procedures, equipment and the use of drugs become
necessary. The authors and the publishers have, as far
as it is possible, taken care to ensure that the
information given in this text is accurate and up to date.
However, readers are strongly advised to confirm that
the information, especially with regard to drug usage,
complies with current legislation and standards of
practice.

The authors wish to record their collaboration with
Dr. John F. Stokes in the production of the first two
editions of this book.

The
publisher's
policy is to use
**paper manufactured
from sustainable forests**

Printed and bound in India

41682 (1)

Self Assessment in Clinical Pharmacology

WARNING

If this book is returned defaced you will be liable to pay for a replacement copy

10|99

04 JAN 2000

03. FEB 09.

24. FEB 09.

03. MAR 09.

29 OCT 19

07 Sep 20

25 Sept

QV18 LAU

For Churchill Livingstone:

Commissioning Editor: Timothy Horne
Project Editor: Janice Urquhart
Project Controller: Frances Affleck
Design direction: Erik Bigland

Preface

This is a book of self assessment questions based on *Clinical Pharmacology* (8th edition) by D. R. Laurence, P. N. Bennett and M. J. Brown. Its objective is to help medical students and postgraduates to pass examinations in clinical pharmacology.

We are, in principle, in favour of such examinations because we think knowledge of drugs and medicines is essential to the competent practice of medicine. Patients are entitled to expect competence from their physician, and physicians owe to their patients a duty of care.

To answer questions is the surest way of finding out whether you know a subject. That some examinations and questions are ill-suited to their purpose does not nullify the principle. *The easiest and the best way to pass an examination is to know its subject.*

It is too easy to read a book and to assume that this has been a profitable exertion. But too often it has not been so. The best assurance that reading has been profitable is to be required or to require oneself to *use* what has been read.

A convenient, quick and private way of doing this is to test yourself with multiple choice questions. Errors teach, if it is possible at once to verify them in an appropriate text; otherwise frustration is the result.

Although *more experienced users* may attempt the questions as they stand, with the object of testing the range of their knowledge, *less experienced* may prefer to read a chapter of the book, and after an interval of some hours, try to answer the questions in this volume. Wrong choices are best checked with the book as they are made, since the purpose is to learn, not merely to record a score.

In almost all cases the correct answer will be found either explicitly or by obvious implication in the text of the chapter being studied, but occasionally reference to another chapter will be needed. Drugs may feature in more that one chapter (e.g. β-adrenoceptor blocking agents) and, when a principle of pharmacokinetics or an adverse reaction is involved, chapters 7 and 8 will repay study. Use of the index is seldom needed, though educationally it is no bad thing to have to search beyong a single chapter for an answer.

Some of the questions are inevitably based on simple memory of facts, the building blocks of pharmacology and medicine. But, in producing these questions we have tried not only to inform and remind but also to illustrate principles. It will be found therefore, that many apparently factual questions can be answered from knowledge of principles. (Principle = fundamental truth as a basis for reasoning: OED.)

Questions are all of the familiar multiple True/False type in which any number of choices within each question may be correct.

1999

D.R.L.
P.N.B.
M.J.B.

Contents

1. Topics in drug therapy   1
2. Clinical pharmacology   9
3. Discovery and development of drugs   11
4. Evaluation of drugs in man   13
5. Official regulation of medicines   21
6. Classification and naming of drugs   25
7. General pharmacology   27
8. Unwanted effects and adverse reactions   41
9. Poisoning, overdose, antidotes   49
10. Nonmedical use of drugs   53
11. Chemotherapy of infections   63
12. Antibacterial drugs   67
13. Chemotherapy of bacterial infections   71
14. Viral, fungal, protozoal and helminthic infections   77
15. Inflammation, arthritis and nonsteroidal anti-inflammatory drugs (NSAIDs)   81
16. Drugs and the skin   85
17. Pain and analgesics   91
18. Sleep and anxiety   99
19. Drugs and mental disorder   103
20. Epilepsy, parkinsonism and allied conditions   111
21. Anaesthesia and neuromuscular block   117
22. Cholinergic and antimuscarinic (anticholinergic) drugs   125

23. Adrenergic mechanisms (sympathomimetics, shock, hypotension) 129

24. Arterial hypertension, angina pectoris, myocardial infarction 133

25. Cardiac dysrhythmia and failure 141

26. Hyperlipidaemias 147

27. Kidney and urinary tract 149

28. Respiratory system 157

29. Drugs and haemostasis 163

30. Cellular disorders and anaemias 169

31. Neoplastic disease and immunosuppression 173

32. Stomach and oesophagus 179

33. Intestines 183

34. Liver, biliary tract, pancreas 187

35. Adrenal corticosteroids, antagonists, corticotrophin 189

36. Diabetes mellitus, insulin, oral antidiabetes agents 197

37. Thyroid hormones, antithyroid drugs 203

38. Hypothalamic, pituitary and sex hormones 207

39. Vitamins, calcium, bone 213

Answers 217

1 Topics in Drug Therapy

1.1   In drug therapy, the following statements are correct:

A   Efficacy and safety of a drug lie solely in its chemical nature
B   Considerations of pharmacokinetics are important
C   Drugs are the major causative factor in the decline of mortality from infectious diseases of the past 100 years
D   The concept of benefit versus risk is central to proper practice
E   Whenever a drug is given a risk is taken

1.2   Disease may be

A   cured by a course of a drug
B   suppressed or controlled, without cure, by a drug
C   prevented by a drug
D   worsened by a drug
E   mimicked by a drug

1.3   Iatrogenic disease

A   occurs as a result of self-medication
B   occurs as a result of prescribed medication
C   is far from rare
D   may result from bad medical advice
E   may be the result of patient noncompliance with clear instructions

1.4   Risk

A   may be graded as unacceptable, acceptable or negligible
B   involved in using penicillin is such that it should only be used in life-endangering infections
C   if unnecessary, is avoided by most people in their daily lives
D   is ignored by most people if it is less than 1:100 000
E   of death from a drug contraindicates its use

1.5   Modern synthetic drugs

A   should not be used until a firm aetiological diagnosis has been made
B   benefit the quality of life more than they do its quantity (duration)
C   are toxic because they are synthetic, not natural, chemicals
D   can only be evaluated by strict randomised controlled trials
E   are only acceptable for use in therapeutics if their mode of action is known

1.6   The following statements about non-scientific, unorthodox medical systems and traditional medicine are correct:

A   Of the terms alternative, fringe and complementary medicine, the term complementary is preferred
B   Traditional or indigenous (prescientific) medical systems have provided no drugs that have stood the test of scientific evaluation
C   Beliefs that cannot be disproved by scientific testing are a feature of unorthodox medical systems
D   Scientific evaluation of unorthodox medical systems is inherently impracticable
E   Iatrogenic disease does not occur in traditional medicine

1.7   The following statements comply with homoeopathic beliefs or practice:

A   Only one disease can exist in the body at any one time

B   Natural disease is cured by introducing into the body by means of a medicine, an artificial disease, which drives out the natural disease

C   The effects of drugs are potentiated by dilution provided each dose contains at least one molecule of drug

D   By shaking a medicine correctly 'a spiritual' therapeutic energy is released

E   If homoeopathic principles (beliefs) cannot be substantiated, i.e. tested and confirmed by use of scientific method, then homoeopathic treatments cannot work

1.8   The following statements about liability for adverse effects of drugs are correct:

A   Liability to compensate for injury of another person caused by negligence (fault) is usual in all legal systems

B   If a patient suffers an adverse drug reaction, someone (the producer or prescriber, for instance) has been negligent

C   It is easy to determine whether an adverse event or worsening of health is due to a drug

D   Some adverse drug reactions could as readily be said to be due to a 'defect' in the patient as to a 'defect' in the drug

E   Capacity to cause harm is inherent in even the most useful drugs

1.9 Despite the manifest difficulties of providing special compensation for drug-caused injury, a scheme to meet public demand might be found socially and politically acceptable if it incorporated the following concepts:

A Liability for drugs under trial before being licensed for general use should fall on the producer

B Liability for recently licensed (by an official regulatory body) drugs may reasonably be shared between the producer and the community (government)

C Liability for standard drugs should fall on a central fund

D Compensation in the case of standard drugs should only be for rare serious effects not ordinarily taken into account when prescribing the drug

E Prolonged legal argument may have to be accepted in cases of compensation for the effects of standard drugs

1.10 The following statements about warnings to patients are correct:

A Doctors do no more than frighten patients by warning them of adverse effects of drugs

B Doctors have a legal duty to warn patients of risks to the extent that in the doctors' judgement is compatible with the particular patient's welfare

C If patients experience adverse reactions of which they were not warned then doctors will be convicted of negligence

D Since patients have died of the consequences of venepuncture, anyone asked to undergo the procedure should be told this fact before deciding whether to agree

E If a patient expresses a wish to leave all considerations of risks of treatment to the doctor, the doctor should yet insist on telling the patient of these risks

1.11 Drug therapy carries risk

A because drugs are not sufficiently selective

B which has been reduced by the development of target-selective carriers such as antibodies

C because patients are homogeneous

D because patients unpredictably develop allergy to drugs

E because dosage adjustment is unavoidably imprecise

1.12 **When taking a patient's history special enquiry should be made about previous use of medicines or other drugs because**

A drugs can cause disease
B withdrawal of drugs can cause disease
C drugs can interact with each other
D drugs can leave residual effects after administration and withdrawal
E knowledge of drug history assists choice of medication in the future

1.13 **Repeat prescriptions in general practice (primary care) are provided by doctors**

A only after personal discussion with the patient
B as a way of terminating the consultation
C as a way of maintaining a relationship
D when they cannot think of anything better to do
E for a patient whose health depends on the specific pharmacological effect of the drug

1.14 **The following statements or opinions about economics in medicine are correct:**

A There are two countries in the world that have enough resources to meet all their citizens' demands for medical care
B Health care cannot be rationed and attempts to do so should not be made
C Cost-effectiveness analysis is a broader activity than is cost–benefit analysis
D Doctors should think only of their patients' immediate personal needs, should fight for these and should not allow economic considerations to intrude
E All expenditure of resources carries a cost in benefits foregone elsewhere, i.e. 'opportunity cost'

1.15 The following statements about drug therapy are correct:

A   The response in acute infections is much influenced by the interaction of the personalities of doctor and patient

B   The response in anxiety or depression is primarily determined by the choice of drug and has little to do with the personal interaction of doctor, patient and social environment

C   Response to a drug can be significantly affected by the initial level of activity of the target organ or system

D   It is of no consequence what sort of medicine the patient thinks he has been given, all that matters is what he has in fact been given

E   Knowledge of why a patient gets better is of purely academic interest

1.16 A placebo effect

A   may follow treatment of all kinds

B   only occurs in mentally ill patients

C   in the individual is an inconstant attribute

D   can be expected in about 35% of patients

E   following a tonic usually has a distinct pharmacological basis

1.17 Placebo reactors tend to be

A   introverted

B   unsociable

C   acquiescent

D   lacking in self-confidence

E   neurotic

1.18 The quality of life of a patient can be assessed by using questionnaires that record, amongst other things,

A   social interaction

B   physical mobility

C   presence of pain

D   capacity for work

E   general well-being

1.19 **Factors established as being associated with patient non-compliance include**

A lack of understanding of instructions
B psychiatric illness
C more than three administration occasions per day
D gender
E family instability

1.20 **The following statements about prescription and administration of drugs in hospital are correct:**

A The concept of compliance applies to patients but not to doctors
B If doctors wrote cheques on their bank accounts as badly as they commonly write prescriptions they would soon be in trouble
C Errors in drug administration in hospitals have been found to occur in about 20% of cases
D Giving physicians information on drugs improves prescribing substantially
E Asking physicians to justify their prescriptions has no effect except to annoy them

1.21 **The following statements about prescribing are correct:**

A Directly observed therapy (DOT) is cheap and convenient
B Fear of being blamed for adverse reactions is one reason why doctors underprescribe
C Drugs do not cause false results in laboratory tests
D The number and cost of prescriptions per head of the population declines after the age of 65 years
E The World Health Organization model list of essential drugs provides a basis for delivering economically affordable health care to the majority of populations

1.22 **The following statements about prescribing are correct:**

A The World Health Organization model list of essential drugs comprises about 750 drugs

B Most doctors manage to do their prescribing from about 100 drugs/formulations

C Generic substitution and therapeutic substitution are cost-containment measures

D 'Appropriate' prescribing means putting considerations of cost first

E The prescribing frequency and costs of younger doctors are higher than those of older doctors, and patients are better off for this

1.23 **Self-medication**

A is an important subject of enquiry when taking a drug history from a patient

B should be permitted only for short-term relief of symptoms

C may be extended to self-management of prescribed drugs in uncomplicated chronic and recurrent diseases

D should have a supply of printed information as a major factor for safety

E is acceptable practice only if the supplier is legally liable for any adverse consequences

2 Clinical pharmacology

2.1 Clinical pharmacology, the scientific study of drugs in man

A is a discipline called into existence by need
B comprises pharmacodynamics, pharmacokinetics, formal therapeutic trials and surveillance studies
C has now become so complex that it can only be conducted by specialist clinical pharmacologists
D poses special ethical and practical limitations
E is fundamentally different from basic pharmacological science conducted on non-human animals or tissues

3 Discovery and development of drugs

3.1 **The discovery of new drugs**

A is an exercise in prediction from studies in animals or tissues, of potential efficacy and safety in humans

B is an exercise in biological selectivity and dose response

C requires demonstration of efficacy in animal models of human disease

D involves the modification of molecular structure of natural chemical mediators as well as of other substances

E requires that a drug intended for long-term use in humans shall undergo life-long general toxicology studies in animals as well as special tests for carcinogenicity and on reproductive function

3.2 **The following statements about pre-clinical drug studies in animals are correct:**

A Establishing the molecular mode of action is a high priority

B Experiments in whole animals have no predictive value for humans

C The principal reason for retaining whole animal studies is that they are cheap to do

D Reproduction studies in animals detect injury to the fetus, but not effects on fertility

E No new drug should be administered to humans until carcinogenicity studies have been completed

3.3 **The following statements about orphan drugs and diseases are correct:**

A An orphan drug is a drug that is therapeutically effective but too toxic for routine use

B An orphan drug is a drug that, for economic reasons, is not developed into a useable medicine

C An orphan disease is a disease that does not respond to therapy

D An orphan disease is a disease so rare that, for economic reasons, therapy is unresearched

E Common diseases in poor communities may also be orphan diseases

4 Evaluation of drugs in man

4.1 Rational development of a potential new drug comprises

A pharmacodynamic and pharmacokinetic studies on healthy subjects or patients

B use on patients to detect potential therapeutic utility

C formal controlled trials

D monitoring for adverse reactions (and efficacy) after release for general prescribing

E the submission of research studies in man to an ethics review committee

4.2 Regulatory guidelines for introduction of a new drug

A require evidence of bioavailability of a formulation

B do not require studies on interaction with other drugs

C state that at least one ingredient of a fixed-dose combination must be relevant to the patient's need

D require that a proprietary product be accompanied by a Data (information) Sheet

E ordinarily require at least three independent therapeutic trials to support a licence application for general use

4.3 **The following statements about the evaluation in man of new drugs are correct:**

A   A new drug should only be tested in man if animal experiments predict a clear advantage

B   All useful drug actions can be demonstrated in healthy volunteers

C   Drug studies in humans where there is no possibility of benefit to the subject are an accepted part of the early process of developing new drugs

D   Bioavailability and bioequivalence are the same thing

E   Good practice requires that patients who have not completed a drug trial regimen be excluded from the final analysis

4.4 **Formal therapeutic trials are particularly efficient at detecting**

A   rare adverse drug effects

B   the efficacy of a drug in uncomplicated disease of mild to moderate severity

C   effects in pregnant women

D   unexpected therapeutic actions

E   drug interactions

4.5 **In the clinical evaluation of therapy the following statements are correct:**

A   Physicians who follow their judgement aided only by personal experience and intuition are not engaging in experiments

B   A scientific experimental approach to therapeutics is inherently less ethical than practice guided by clinical experience and impression

C   General impressions are never to be trusted

D   The general principles need not concern practising doctors

E   If a patient gets better after treatment it is reasonable to conclude that the recovery is due to the treatment

4.6   Therapeutic trials are designed to show as far as is practicable

A   whether a treatment is of value
B   how great is its value
C   in what type of patients it is of value
D   what is the best method of applying the treatment
E   what are the disadvantages or dangers of a treatment

4.7   Features of the classic randomised controlled therapeutic trial include

A   precisely framed question to be answered
B   equivalent groups of patients
C   groups formed by allocating alternate patients to each treatment under investigation
D   treatments carried out concurrently
E   double-blind technique where evaluation depends on strictly objective measurements

4.8   Placebo or dummy medication

A   provides a control device by which true pharmacodynamic effects of therapy are distinguished from the general psychological effects of medication
B   provides a device to avoid false negative conclusions
C   is inherently unethical
D   is always scientifically necessary in a trial of drug therapy
E   is sometimes used in patients who also receive a pharmacologically active treatment

4.9   In a therapeutic trial

A   different active treatments must never be given to the same patient

B   the order in which treatments are given may influence the results

C   the theoretical basis of the design is to test the hypothesis that there is no difference between the treatments under test

D   there is a risk of finding a difference where there is in reality no difference

E   there is no risk of finding no difference where there is in reality a difference

4.10   A statistical significance test

A   is a device concerned with probabilities rather than with certainties

B   when negative is of little interest unless the confidence interval is also stated and is narrow

C   plus a statement of confidence interval helps to avoid a Type 1 error

D   cannot be of use in cross-over studies

E   showing $P = 0.05$ means that if the experiment were repeated 100 times, there being in reality no difference between the treatments, then a difference as great as that observed would occur 5 times as a result of chance

4.11 Statisticians

A   can salvage a poorly designed experiment after it has been completed

B   cannot tell clinicians how many patients they will need in a therapeutic trial to get a clinically important result unless clinicians can be explicit on the differences they expect and the risk they are prepared to accept of getting a misleading result (Type I error, Type II error)

C   contributes both to the precision of a therapeutic experiment and to its ethics

D   can prove that differences between treatments are clinically important

E   is likely to advise that a simple significance test conducted at regular intervals, the trial ceasing as soon as a positive result is obtained, is the best way of deciding when to stop a trial

4.12 The following statements about therapeutic trials are correct:

A   Knowledge of the results of a therapeutic trial conducted in groups of patients does not help the physician faced with an individual patient

B   A clinician who is personally convinced that treatment A is better than treatment B cannot ethically engage in a scientific study on the subject

C   Once a therapeutic trial has given a positive result it becomes unethical to do another similar trial

D   To conduct a scientific study in which the patient's treatment is chosen by random allocation is inherently unethical

E   A good guide to conduct is that no patient participating in a therapeutic trial should be worse off than he or she might otherwise have been in the hands of a competent doctor

4.13 The following statements about therapeutic trials are correct:

A Numbers of patients in trial groups must be equal or as nearly equal as possible

B Surrogate effects may be used

C To collect all published studies and analyse them together was a good idea but it has proved scientifically unworkable because of publication bias

D Where large formal therapeutic trials are logistically impracticable large observational studies of patients treated in the ordinary way of practice are better than nothing

E Clinical specialists are slower to implement in their practice the results of therapeutic trials than are nonspecialists

4.14 A case control study

A involves a retrospective approach and thus is inherently less valid scientifically than a prospective study such as the randomised controlled trial

B reveals associations but does not prove causation

C involves collecting a control group of subjects similar in essentials but without the condition under study

D involves taking a drug history from each subject in order to compare the incidence of consumption (in each group) of the drug under suspicion (of an adverse effect)

E gives results quicker than does an observational cohort study

4.15 The following statements about relative and absolute risk in therapeutic and preventive trials are correct:

A   A change in clinical outcome (benefit or risk) from 2% to 1% is a 50% change

B   A change in clinical outcome (benefit or risk) from 2% to 1% means that it is necessary to treat 100 patients to provide benefit to one patient

C   Practising clinicians need to know how many patients must be exposed to a drug to achieve one desired outcome

D   A statement of relative risk reduction in preventive trials tells clinicians as much as they need to know about risk

E   Knowledge of absolute risk is particularly important in studies of the prevention of low-incidence clinical events

5 Official regulation of medicines

5.1 **The following statements about official drug regulation and its history are correct:**

A Modern comprehensive official drug regulation began in the USA (1938) after an accident involving sulphanilamide and diethylene glycol

B The company making the mixture tested it for fragrance and flavour but not for safety

C The lack of testing for safety did not infringe the then law in the USA

D The rest of the world only accepted the need for comprehensive control following the thalidomide disaster (1961)

E No new drug should be licensed for general prescribing (marketed) until it has been proved unable to do harm

5.2 **Official drug regulation or control is concerned with**

A quality of the manufactured drug and formulation

B safety of the drug

C efficacy of the drug

D supply to the medical profession and the public

E compiling a register of accepted medicinal products

5.3 **A modern effective drug regulatory authority requires evidence derived from**

A studies on animals

B chemical and pharmaceutical quality studies

C pharmacological studies in man

D formal therapeutic trials

E post-licensing (marketing) surveillance

5.4   The following statements are correct:

A   There are risks in taking drugs
B   There are no risks in not taking drugs
C   Safety of a drug means safety in relation to its clinical use
D   The earliest stage of new drug testing in humans is normally performed in males
E   It is harder to detect and quantitate a harm that is done than it is to detect a good that is not done

5.5   The following statements are correct:

A   Drugs may have an environmental impact
B   A licence to market a new drug should be for an indefinite period
C   Post-licensing surveillance should be unnecessary if the regulatory authority has done its job properly
D   Licence to market a new drug should be witheld until the developer has demonstrated, by comparative clinical studies, that the drug is better than existing drugs, i.e. is needed in medicine
E   Doctors may not prescribe a drug for an unlicensed use

5.6   Drug regulators

A   should not take risks on behalf of society
B   face uncertainty as to the true facts about a new drug at the time when they are required to decide whether or not to grant a licence for general use
C   are in the business of taking simple scientific decisions based on the evidence submitted to them
D   are not prone to defensive practices
E   could well have as a motto, 'It seemed the right thing to do at the time'

5.7 **The following statements about thalidomide and the thalidomide disaster are correct:**

A   Tests on pregnant animals had been done before marketing

B   Thalidomide caused major anatomical abnormalities in fetuses when taken by the mother in the final six weeks of pregnancy

C   Thalidomide still remains in restricted clinical use

D   Thalidomide was recognised as harmful to human fetuses as soon as it was because it caused a very severe effect that was ordinarily seen extremely rarely

E   When thalidomide was first suspected a case-control study was quickly done

6 Classification and naming of drugs

6.1 **The following statements are correct:**

A Classification is a fundamental requirement of a science
B Nomenclature is a fundamental requirement of science
C A drug or medicine generally has three names
D Proprietary names apply to pure drug substances rather than to formulations
E There is a single classification of drugs that suits all interested parties

6.2 **Drugs are generally classified by their**

A proprietary names
B adverse effects
C mode of action
D molecular structure
E therapeutic use

6.3 **The following statements about nomenclature of drugs are correct:**

A Proprietary names are chosen to emphasise the similarities between similar drugs
B Official (nonproprietary) names are chosen to emphasise the differences between related drugs
C The full chemical name is best for prescribing purposes
D There is never a medically important reason for using a proprietary name in prescribing
E The majority of mixed formulations of drugs do not have nonproprietary names

7 General pharmacology

7.1 Drugs may act

A through enzyme inhibition
B by being incorporated into larger molecules
C outside the cell
D by chelation
E by osmotic effect

7.2 The following statements about drug action on cell membranes are correct:

A Antihistamines act on specific receptors
B Volatile anaesthetics act on specific receptors
C Cardiac antidysrhythmia drugs interfere with selective passage of ions
D Drugs may act through membrane-bound enzymes
E Drugs act on cell membrane constituents themselves

7.3 The following statements about drugs and receptors are correct:

A Agonists exert their principal effect by blockading receptors
B Antagonists exert their principal effect by activating receptors
C Inverse agonists produce effects that are specifically opposite to those of the agonist
D Propranolol has partial agonist activity
E Phenoxybenzamine binds irreversibly to the α-adrenoceptor

7.4 Competitive antagonism

A can be reversed by increasing the amount of agonist present

B to agonist alone is not parallel to the curve obtained when an antagonist is present

C is exemplified by the use of ethanol in methanol poisoning

D never occurs with enzymes

E is the same as physiological antagonism

7.5 The following drugs act principally by inhibiting enzymes:

A Enalapril

B Carbidopa

C Aspirin

D Atropine in the management of overdose with a beta-blocker

E Adrenaline in anaphylactic shock

7.6 The following statements about dose and response are correct:

A The dose-response curves of loop diuretics rapidly reach a plateau

B Thiazide diuretics have a steep and prolonged dose-response curve

C If one drug has greater therapeutic efficacy than another then it is more potent

D If one drug is more potent than another drug then it can achieve a therapeutic effect of greater magnitude

E The therapeutic index is the maximum tolerated dose divided by the minimum curative dose

7.7   The following statements about the order of drug metabolic reaction processes are correct:

A   Processes for which rate is proportional to concentration are termed first-order
B   Processes for which the rate is constant regardless of changes in concentration are termed zero-order
C   First-order processes exhibit saturation kinetics
D   Alcohol in 'social' doses is metabolised by a zero-order process
E   Phenytoin is eliminated by first-order processes throughout the clinical dose range

7.8   First-order processes

A   apply only to enzyme-mediated processes
B   proceed at high rates when the concentrations of substances are high and vice versa
C   can properly be described in terms of $t_{\frac{1}{2}}$
D   apply to most drugs in clinical use
E   apply to salicylate metabolism throughout the therapeutic dose range

7.9   In zero-order kinetics

A   elimination rate is independent of dose
B   the $t_{\frac{1}{2}}$ is constant despite rising drug concentration
C   enzyme-mediated metabolic reactions become saturated
D   uniform increases in dose may result in disproportionate increases in plasma concentration
E   passive diffusion processes become saturated

7.10 **The following statements about drugs eliminated by first-order processes are correct:**

A A drug of $t_\frac{1}{2}$ 6 h that is present in the plasma at a steady concentration of 100 mg/l will have a concentration of 25 mg/l 18 h after administration is discontinued

B A drug having a $t_\frac{1}{2}$ of 6 h will, after 12 h, attain a plasma concentration that is 75% of the ultimate steady-state concentration

C The time for a drug to reach steady-state concentration in plasma is a function only of $t_\frac{1}{2}$

D When a drug is at steady-state concentration in plasma and a different, regularly administered, dose is given, a new steady-state concentration will be attained in two $t_\frac{1}{2}$s

E A drug that is given by repeated oral administration can be said to have reached steady-state concentration in plasma when all peaks are of equal height

7.11 **The $t_\frac{1}{2}$ of**

A benzylpenicillin is 30 minutes
B atenolol is 24 hours
C digoxin is 36 hours
D dobutamine is 2 minutes
E piroxicam is 45 hours

7.12 **Drug plasma concentration measurements are not of practical use in the case of**

A oral anticoagulants
B diuretics
C monoamine oxidase inhibitors
D treatment with lithium
E hypoglycaemics

7.13 **Factors that make it difficult to establish correlation between drug plasma concentration and pharmacological effect include**

A the presence in the plasma of pharmacologically active metabolites

B the use of an assay technique that measures pharmacologically inactive metabolites

C the use of an assay technique that measures total (bound + free) drug in plasma

D the presence of a 'therapeutic window'

E the irreversible action of 'hit and run' drugs

7.14 **Monitoring of plasma concentration of drugs is a useful guide to therapy**

A in some cases of cardiac dysrhythmia

B in some cases of drug overdose

C with aminoglycoside antibiotics

D irrespective of the timing of blood sampling in relation to that of dosing

E for drugs with low therapeutic index

7.15 **Passage of drug across cell membranes**

A by diffusion requires cellular energy

B by diffusion exhibits first-order kinetics

C by filtration is most readily accomplished by neutral (uncharged) molecules

D by filtration occurs at the renal glomerulus

E by active transport may involve competition with other molecules of similar structure

7.16 **The following statements about passage of drugs across cell membranes are correct:**

A   Un-ionised drug is lipid soluble and diffusible
B   The acidic environment of the stomach favours absorption of aspirin from that site
C   Atenolol (water soluble) enters the CNS more readily than propranolol (lipid soluble)
D   Polar (permanently charged) drugs readily cross cell membranes
E   Levodopa is actively transported across the blood–brain barrier

7.17 **The following statements about drug ionisation are correct:**

A   Acidic groups become less ionised in an acid medium
B   The pKa is the negative logarithm of the Ka (ionisation constant)
C   Some drugs are incapable of becoming ionised
D   The pKa varies with environmental pH
E   Many drugs are weak electrolytes

7.18 **The following statements about drug absorption from the gastrointestinal tract are correct:**

A   The buccal route of administration gives rapid effect because mucosal blood flow is abundant
B   The stomach is a major site of drug absorption
C   The rate of gastric emptying can have a major influence on drug absorption
D   Enterohepatic recycling helps to retain oral contraceptive steroids in the body
E   The colon is incapable of absorbing drugs

7.19 Bioavailability

A refers to the amount of drug that is released from a dose form

B is highly dependent on the size of the particles of which a tablet is made

C is influenced by diluting substances within a dose form

D of different formulations is demonstrated by measuring plasma concentration-time profiles following administration of the same dose to individuals one after another

E differences may be the cause of unexpected drug toxicity or failure of therapy

7.20 Presystemic elimination

A may account for differences in enteral and parenteral drug dosages that achieve comparable effect

B is significant in the case of morphine administered by the oral route

C is significant in the case of chlormethiazole administered by the oral route

D is significant in the case of pethidine administered by the oral route

E may be reduced if the liver is diseased

7.21 Enteral administration

A of a drug may result in reduced absorption after food

B of gentamicin is the preferred route for systemic effect

C of solid dose forms should ideally take place lying down

D of a drug by the buccal route can be terminated rapidly

E of sustained-release potassium chloride may cause oesophageal ulceration

7.22 Rectal administration of drugs

A always provides reliable effects

B completely avoids first-pass elimination

C may be useful in migraine

D may cause proctitis

E is useful for drugs that irritate the stomach

7.23 Parenteral administration of a drug

A by the intravenous route may need to take account of the rate of blood circulation

B to the eye may cause systemic effects

C by intramuscular injection results in slower absorption than by subcutaneous injection

D by inhalation is used only for local effect in the lung

E through the skin may give a reliable systemic effect

7.24 The apparent distribution volume of a drug

A is the volume of fluid in which it appears to distribute with a concentration equal to that in plasma

B is small if it remains in the plasma

C normally corresponds precisely with a physiological space such as extracellular water

D cannot exceed total body volume

E is determined by dividing the dose given by the estimated concentration at zero time after an intravenous bolus injection

7.25 On the basis of apparent volume of distribution, haemodialysis would be effective in removing drug from subjects overdosed with

A chloroquine

B pethidine

C salicylate

D digoxin

E nortriptyline

7.26 The following statements about drug binding to plasma proteins and tissues are correct:

A Bound drug is pharmacologically active

B The main binding protein for many drugs is albumin

C Drug protein binding may be reduced in chronic renal disease

D Extensive tissue binding delays the elimination of chloroquine

E Quinidine and digoxin compete for binding sites in tissues

7.27   Drug distribution may be influenced by

A   body fluid pH
B   regional blood flow
C   plasma protein binding
D   lipid solubility
E   binding to body tissues

7.28   Drug metabolism

A   generally results in metabolites having increased lipid solubility
B   generally converts a pharmacologically active to an inactive substance
C   in the case of amitriptyline converts a pharmacologically active substance to another active substance
D   in the case of enalapril converts a pharmacologically inactive substance to an active substance
E   by conjugation normally terminates biological activity

7.29   Enzyme induction

A   with antiepilepsy drugs may cause osteomalacia
B   contributes to tolerance to the acute effects of alcohol
C   enables the body to adapt to varying exposure to foreign compounds
D   renders patients less susceptible to effects of paracetamol overdose
E   may be a cause of failure of oral contraception

7.30   Enzyme induction

A   may be caused by rifampicin
B   may occur with a diet that includes barbecued meats and Brussels sprouts
C   may be a cause of failure of anticoagulant control with warfarin
D   caused by heavy alcohol consumption may be a cause of failure of expected drug response
E   is not caused by tobacco smoke

7.31 Enzyme inhibition

A due to cimetidine reduces the effects of concurrently administered theophylline

B due to allopurinol is used in the treatment of alcoholism

C due to enalapril is used in the treatment of hypertension

D due to monoamine oxidase inhibitors increases the effect of some sympathomimetics

E due to sodium valproate increases the effect of phenytoin

7.32 The following statements about drugs in breast milk are correct:

A Loss in milk is a significant mechanism of elimination from the body

B Anticancer drugs may safely be given to breastfeeding mothers

C Most drugs taken by the mother pose no hazard to the suckling child

D Use of aminophylline by a breast feeding mother may cause her infant to become irritable

E Use of antiepilepsy drugs may cause the infant to become sedated

7.33 The following statements about drug elimination are correct:

A Renal clearance of a drug that is eliminated only by filtration by the kidney cannot exceed the glomerular filtration rate

B In general, biliary excretion is limited to substances with molecular weight >300

C The high renal clearance of benzylpenicillin indicates that this drug is secreted by the renal tubules

D Substances having a molecular weight of 10 000 are excluded from the glomerular filtrate

E Alkalinisation of the urine is used to increase the renal clearance of salicylate in overdose

7.34 The following statements about drug dosing are correct:

A For a drug with a $t_{\frac{1}{2}}$ of >24 h, the daily maintenance must be arranged to equal the amount of drug that leaves the body in 24 h

B For a drug with a $t_{\frac{1}{2}}$ of <3 h, administering half the priming dose at intervals equal to the $t_{\frac{1}{2}}$ is an acceptable regimen

C Drugs with long $t_{\frac{1}{2}}$ are especially suitable for administration as sustained release preparations

D Combining a drug injected s.c. with adrenaline can be expected to shorten its duration of action

E Probenecid accelerates the excretion of penicillin

7.35 Fixed-dose drug combinations

A are appropriate for the treatment of tuberculosis

B are appropriate for the treatment of Parkinson's disease

C are appropriate for drugs with a wide range of dose

D may facilitate compliance with medication in the elderly

E may render difficult the identification of adverse reactions

7.36 Long-term use

A of drugs may be associated with resurgence of disease when drug is withdrawn

B of β-adrenoceptor agonists is associated with receptor up-regulation

C of benzodiazepines, followed by abrupt discontinuation, is safe

D of β-adrenoceptor antagonists is associated with adverse effects if discontinuation is abrupt

E of drugs may mask progression of disease

7.37 Genetic variation

A may explain lack of response to normal doses of warfarin

B may be the cause of vitamin D-resistant rickets

C may be the cause of adverse reaction to dapsone

D that is discontinuous is due to a single gene effect, i.e. is monofactorial

E may explain failure to breathe after a surgical operation

7.38 **The following statements about age and drugs are correct:**

A Drugs are readily absorbed through the skin of the infant
B Distribution of drugs in the neonate is influenced by the lower proportion of fat and the higher proportion of water
C Drug metabolism is especially slow in the neonate
D Serum creatinine is a reliable indicator of the capacity to eliminate drugs by the kidney in the elderly
E Drugs that act on the nervous system have reduced effect in the elderly

7.39 **Pharmacokinetics may be influenced by**

A pregnancy
B migraine
C resection and reconstruction of the gut
D chronic liver disease
E severe cardiac failure

7.40 **Interaction between drugs**

A with steep dose-response curves is unlikely to be harmful
B with small therapeutic ratios is unlikely to be harmful
C is described as summation if the effects of two drugs having the same action are additive
D is described as potentiation if the action of one drug increases the effect of another
E may lead to valuable therapeutic effects

7.41 **Interactions of drugs in the gut may be**

A due to altered motility
B the result of purgation
C due to direct chemical reaction
D due to alteration of gut flora
E avoided by separating doses by 2 hours

7.42   Drug interaction between

A   naloxone and morphine occurs primarily at plasma protein binding sites

B   rifampicin and cyclosporin may lead to cyclosporin toxicity

C   quinolone antimicrobials and theophylline may lead to loss of efficacy of theophylline

D   lithium and a thiazide diuretic may cause lithium toxicity

E   phenytoin and the oral contraceptive pill may lead to pregnancy

7.43   The following statements about interactions between drugs are correct:

A   Drugs classed as monoamine oxidase (A+B) inhibitors alter clinical responses only to sympathomimetics

B   Metronidazole alters the clinical effects of alcohol

C   Allopurinol inhibits azathioprine metabolism, with risk of toxicity

D   Nonsteroidal anti-inflammatory drugs may cause loss of antihypertensive control with β-adrenoceptor blockers

E   Probenecid accelerates the renal elimination of penicillin

7.44   Clinically important interactions between drugs

A   take place only in the body

B   can occur only when drugs have the same site of action

C   are invariably harmful

D   may be antagonistic

E   may result in potentiation of effect

8 Unwanted effects and adverse drug reactions

8.1 **The following statements about unwanted effects of drugs (adverse reactions) are correct:**

A There is a fundamental biological distinction between therapeutic and adverse effects of drugs

B Some adverse effects are due to normal predictable pharmacological effects of drugs and may occur in any patient taking the drug

C Some adverse effects are due to abnormalities in the patient and will only occur in some patients taking the drug

D The terms intolerant and tolerant refer to individuals at either extreme of the normal distribution curve

E Idiosyncrasy means allergy

8.2 **The following statements about adverse drug reaction detection are correct:**

A Formal therapeutic trials reliably detect adverse reactions having an incidence of 1:10 000

B Spontaneous reporting systems provide reliable quantitative data on incidence of adverse reaction

C Drug-induced illness is often similar to spontaneous disease

D When monitoring new drugs recently licensed for general use doctors are asked to report all events which could conceivably be due to the drug

E If it is desired reliably to detect a serious adverse reaction having an incidence of 1:10,000 (and no spontaneous incidence in the community) it will be necessary to monitor about 65 000 patients

8.3 **In investigating the possibility of drug-induced illness the finding that**

A a drug commonly induces an otherwise rare illness is detectable only with the utmost difficulty

B a drug rarely induces an otherwise common illness may go for ever undiscovered

C a drug rarely induces an otherwise rare illness is likely to be detected early in pre-licensing clinical trials

D a drug commonly induces an otherwise common illness is likely to be detected by informal clinical observation

E adverse reactions are a cause will be determined most reliably by clinical observation supported by case control and cohort studies

8.4 **Adverse drug reactions**

A cause 2–3% of consultations in general practice

B cause up to 3% of admissions to acute care hospital wards

C are particularly likely to occur in females over 60 years old

D are more likely to occur late rather than early in therapy

E are a common cause of death following therapeutic use in the UK

8.5 **Adverse drug reactions**

A may be dose-related

B may follow long-term use of neuroleptics

C of the idiosyncratic type account for most fatalities

D are unlikely to follow abrupt discontinuation of drugs

E may affect the next biological generation

8.6 **Factors which may influence the incidence of adverse reactions to drugs include**

A age

B sex

C genetic constitution

D disease

E tendency to allergy

8.7 **Adverse drug reactions may be influenced by**

A inherent properties of the drug
B the length of time for which a drug is used
C discontinuing use of a drug
D the ingredients of the formulation as well as the active drug itself
E other drugs the patient is taking

8.8 **The following statements about adverse drug reactions are correct:**

A Pharmacokinetic mechanisms are unimportant in causation
B Young children can be regarded as 'small adults' as far as liability to adverse drug reactions is concerned
C The first few weeks of life is a period of special risk
D Old age is a period of special risk
E Atmospheric pollution in hospitals may be a cause

8.9 **The elderly show an increased response to standard drug dosage and an increased incidence of adverse drug reactions because they have**

A reduced total body water
B reduced renal and hepatic function
C reduced maximum breathing capacity
D decreased lean body mass
E reduced baroreceptor sensitivity

8.10 **Patients having the following conditions tend to show a greater than normal response to some drugs:**

A Hypoalbuminaemia
B Congestive cardiac failure
C Hepatic cirrhosis
D Hyperthyroidism
E Hypothyroidism

8.11 The following statements about hepatic porphyrias are correct:

A They are characterised by accumulation of porphyrins
B They are due to single gene defects
C Presentation may be as acute illness after medication
D Acute attacks are not provoked by enzyme-inducing drugs
E Acute attacks may usefully be treated with haem arginate

8.12 An attack of porphyria may be precipitated by

A aspirin
B morphine
C phenobarbitone
D carbamazepine
E some 'home remedies', e.g. mouthwash

8.13 The following statements about adverse drug reactions are correct:

A Glaucoma in an asthmatic can safely be treated with β-adrenoceptor eye drops
B A skin rash following use of ampicillin in a patient having a sore throat raises the possibility that the patient has infectious mononucleosis
C In peripheral circulatory failure from any cause drugs should not be injected subcutaneously
D Patients with raised intracranial pressure are intolerant of opioids
E In myasthenia gravis, muscular weakness is made worse by quinidine

8.14 **The following statements about drug allergy are correct:**

A   All drugs are antigens

B   If antibodies to a drug are present in patients, then they will suffer an adverse reaction if they receive the drug again

C   Drugs or drug metabolites combine with a body protein to form an antigen

D   Allergic reactions reproduce, only with greater intensity, the normal pharmacological actions of the causative drug

E   Drugs elicit only Type 1 (immediate or anaphylactic) allergic reactions

8.15 **Where a drug causes an allergic (immunological) illness**

A   it is safe to change to another member of the same chemical class

B   there is no linear relation of dose to effect

C   safe desensitisation is impossible

D   re-exposure to a small dose is enough to cause illness

E   there has been a preceding first exposure followed by an interval

8.16 **Important manifestations of drug allergy include**

A   thrombocytopenia

B   granulocytopenia/agranulocytosis

C   leukaemia

D   aplastic anaemia

E   haemolysis

8.17 **Important direct manifestations of drug allergy include**

A   serum sickness syndrome

B   asthma

C   cardiac dysrhythmia

D   cholestatic jaundice

E   epilepsy

8.18 In drug allergy

A laboratory tests are essential for diagnosis
B intradermal injection tests can cause anaphylactic shock
C patch skin tests give reliable diagnostic information for contact dermatitis only
D detection of drug-specific circulating antibodies is used to establish allergy to penicillin
E once allergy has occurred it is permanent

8.19 Anaphylactic shock is an Immunological condition in which

A interaction of antigen with antibody causes cell damage with release of biologically active substances
B histamine is an important cause of the shock
C the blood pressure falls dramatically
D the bronchi dilate dramatically
E the emergency treatment is adrenaline given intramuscularly followed by a histamine H1-receptor antagonist followed by an adrenocortical steroid

8.20 In drug allergy

A patients should be clearly informed about the drug(s) to which they may react
B desensitisation (hyposensitisation) may be only temporary
C a sensible course is to give a patient another drug from the same chemical group
D reaction may be to ingredients of the formulation
E desensitisation (hyposensitisation) should be undertaken in all patients suspected of penicillin allergy

8.21 In early pregnancy

A drugs may damage the embryo or fetus indirectly by altering the mother's physiology
B ergot alkaloids can cause abortion
C abortion may go unrecognised
D cytotoxics are safe
E teratogens are likely to have their most devastating effects

8.22   In late pregnancy or labour

   A   gross anatomical defects in the fetus are likely to result from drugs

   B   nonsteroidal anti-inflammatory drugs can delay the onset of labour

   C   a vasoconstrictor drug given to the mother can cause fetal distress

   D   opioids given to the mother may depress fetal respiration

   E   benzodiazepines given to the mother do not affect the fetus

8.23   Substances strongly suspected or known to be capable of harming the fetus when consumed by a pregnant woman include

   A   penicillin

   B   sex hormones

   C   phenytoin

   D   warfarin

   E   alcohol

8.24   The following statements concerning teratogenicity are correct:

   A   The concept of absolute drug safety needs to be demolished in the public mind

   B   In real life it can never be shown that a drug (or anything else) has no teratogenic activity at all

   C   When prescribing for a substantial period it is as important to consider whether a woman may become pregnant as whether she is already pregnant

   D   Some drugs in common use may be unrecognised low grade teratogens

   E   Fetal abnormality may be due to the disease for which the drug was prescribed

9 Poisoning, overdose, antidotes

9.1 In self-poisoning

A most cases represent a serious attempt to end life
B alcohol is also taken in over 50% of cases
C there is a mortality rate of about 1% of acute hospital admissions
D accidental episodes occur predominantly amongst children
E repeated episodes are rare

9.2 In acute poisoning

A analysis of plasma is valueless in lithium overdose
B response to flumazenil is valuable in diagnosis for opioid drugs
C analysis of plasma for iron is useful in iron overdose
D naloxone should be used for benzodiazepine overdose
E with carbon tetrachloride, acetylcysteine is of value

9.3 In the treatment of acute poisoning

A both therapeutic emesis and gastric lavage are contraindicated for corrosive poisons
B gastric lavage is of no value more than 5 hours after a tricyclic antidepressant has been taken
C with a β-adrenoceptor antagonist, glucagon may be beneficial
D the active constituent of ipecacuanha can cause drowsiness
E gastric lavage should take place before emergency resuscitation procedures

9.4   In acute poisoning

A   with aspirin, activated charcoal in repeated doses is
     an acceptable treatment
B   acidification of the urine is commonly undertaken
C   peritoneal dialysis is as effective as haemodialysis
D   due to swallowing antifreeze solution haemodialysis is
     ineffective
E   with salicylate, alkalinisation of the urine may form part
     of the treatment

9.5   In the treatment of a patient with drug overdose

A   hypothermia may need to be corrected
B   cardiac dysrhythmia is an indication for immediate use of
     antidysrhythmic drugs
C   a systolic blood pressure of 80 mm Hg may be tolerated
     in a young person
D   rhabdomyolysis is an incidental finding which may be
     ignored
E   diazepam should not be used to treat convulsions

**9.6   The following antidotes and their indications for use in
         poisoning are correctly paired:**

A   Calcium gluconate; indandione anticoagulants
B   Ethanol; methanol
C   Phentolamine; β-adrenoceptor blocking agents
D   Acetylcysteine; paracetamol
E   Atropine; organophosphorus insecticides

9.7   Chelation therapy

A   with dimercaprol is ineffective for arsenic poisoning
B   with dimercaprol is efficacious through the provision of
     -SH chemical groups
C   for severe lead poisoning may require both sodium
     calcium edetate and dimercaprol
D   with penicillamine may be used for hepatolenticular
     degeneration
E   with unithiol (DMPS) is effective for mercury poisoning

9.8   In cyanide poisoning

A   early symptoms are similar to those of anxiety
B   the breath smells of bitter almonds
C   specific treatment is by dicobalt edetate
D   sodium thiosulphate is useful in the later stages of
    treatment
E   treatment differs from that of carbon monoxide poisoning
    in that there is no place for hyperbaric oxygen

9.9   The following statements are correct:

A   Chronic abusers of volatile solvents may develop
    cerebellar disease
B   Methanol poisoning may cause blindness
C   Poisoning with ethylene glycol leads to acidosis
D   In methanol poisoning, peritoneal dialysis is more
    effective than haemodialysis
E   Death from solvent abuse is commonly due to cardiac
    dysrhythmia

**9.10   The following statements about herbicides and
         pesticides are correct:**

A   Dinitro-orthocresol is not absorbed through the skin
B   In poisoning by dinitro-compounds symptoms and signs
    indicate a high metabolic rate
C   Strychnine causes convulsions
D   Paraquat is taken up in the lungs
E   Fuller's earth should be given urgently both in paraquat
    and in diquat poisoning

**9.11   The following statements about poisoning with
         biological substances are correct**

A   Deadly nightshade(*Atropa belladonna*) causes blurred
    vision
B   Laburnum causes salivation
C   Lily-of-the-valley (*Convallaria*) causes cardiac dysrhythmia
D   *Amanita phalloides* (death cap mushroom) is hepatotoxic
E   Liberty cap mushrooms are hallucinogenic

9.12 CS, a common antiriot agent

A is a solid used in particulate aerosol form
B causes persistent bronchospasm even in normal people
C can cause a gripping pain in the chest
D has a plasma $t_{\frac{1}{2}}$ of about 5 seconds
E causes excessive salivation which may persist for an hour

9.13 Drugs which have probably been used for torture or 'interrogation' include

A cyclophosphamide
B amphetamine
C thiopentone
D suxamethonium
E apomorphine

10 Nonmedical use of drugs

10.1   Motives for nonmedical drug use include

A   relief of anxiety and personal psychological problems
B   search for self-knowledge and meaning in life
C   conformity with social subgroup
D   fun, recreation
E   success in sport

10.2   The following statements about nonmedical drug use and drug abuse are correct:

A   Abuse potential of a drug is related to its capacity to produce immediate satisfaction
B   Abuse potential of a drug is uninfluenced by its route of administration
C   Drugs that insulate the individual from environmental stress and anxiety are the most likely to be abused
D   Volatile inhalants tend to be used by those under 16 years of age
E   Surviving users tend to reduce or relinquish heavy use as they enter middle age

10.3 The following statements about nonmedical drug use or abuse are correct:

A Drug abuse implies excessive nonmedical or social drug use

B It is not the drug alone, but also the way it is used that provides the basis for the classification 'hard' and 'soft'

C Spiritual or religious experience can be regarded as a normal dose-related pharmacodynamic effect of some drugs

D The claim that drugs can provide a basis for a 'culture' may best be judged by results, i.e. by the contribution of its exponents to society in terms of practice and example

E Even 'soft' use of drugs such as alcohol and tobacco is so potentially hazardous that it should be countered by legislation designed to eliminate them from society

10.4 The following statements about the use of drugs to gain advantage in sport are correct:

A Anabolic steroids may reduce testosterone production

B Stimulants such as amphetamine are used to improve performance in the 100 m sprint

C β-adrenoceptor blocking drugs may improve performance in pistol shooting

D Diuretics may be used in the hope of avoiding detection of performance enhancing drugs

E Caffeine can improve physical performance

10.5 Features of the drug dependent state include

A emotional distress if the drug is withheld

B physical illness if the drug is withheld

C a need to increase the dose

D continuous use

E intermittent use

10.6 **The following statements about drug dependence and tolerance are correct:**

A   Physical dependence is a major factor with cocaine
B   Physical dependence is a major factor with opioids
C   Cross tolerance between different chemical classes of drug does not occur
D   Cross tolerance occurs between members of the same chemical class of drug
E   Emotional dependence may occur with any drug that alters consciousness

10.7 **Morphine-type drug dependence is characterised by**

A   severe physical dependence
B   slight emotional dependence
C   marked tolerance
D   cross-tolerance with other opioids
E   resistance to naloxone

10.8 **Barbiturate-type drug dependence is characterised by**

A   severe emotional dependence
B   slight physical dependence
C   tolerance
D   cross-tolerance with alcohol
E   cross-tolerance with benzodiazepines

10.9 **The following statements about drug abuse or dependence are correct:**

A   Cannabis induces marked physical dependence and tolerance
B   Tobacco induces severe emotional dependence
C   Amphetamine use can cause a psychotic state
D   Cocaine induces marked tolerance
E   Physical dependence occurs with prolonged heavy use of alcohol

10.10 The following statements about treatment of drug dependence are correct:

A Heroin addiction should be treated with chlordiazepoxide

B Chlormethiazole should be used to manage alcohol withdrawal

C Pentazocine may induce a withdrawal syndrome in opioid addicts

D A variable proportion of subjects who start with cannabis eventually take heroin

E Pulmonary embolism is a complication of illicit i.v. drug use

10.11 The following statements about tobacco smoking are correct:

A Smoke of pipes and cigars is alkaline and therefore nicotine is readily absorbed via the buccal mucosa

B Nicotine is chiefly responsible for the long-term adverse effects of smoking

C Cigarette smokers tend to inhale

D Cigar and pipe smokers tend not to inhale

E Cigarette smokers who inhale may have as much as 15% of their haemoglobin converted to carboxyhaemoglobin

10.12 Pharmacological aspects of tobacco smoking include

A stimulation of the vomiting centre

B tolerance

C increased platelet adhesiveness

D increased airways resistance

E no notable cardiovascular effects

10.13 **The following statements about the risks of tobacco smoking are correct:**

A   15% of male nonsmokers aged 35 years are dead by age 65 years

B   40% of male smokers of 25 or more cigarettes a day are dead by age 65 years

C   Cigarette smoking causes induction of hepatic metabolising enzymes

D   The time by which a habitual smoker's life is shortened is about one hour for each cigarette smoked

E   The higher death rate of smokers is chiefly the result of cardiovascular and respiratory diseases

10.14 **The following statements about smoking and cancer are correct:**

A   Risk of lung cancer is related to the number of cigarettes smoked

B   Risk of lung cancer is related to the age of starting smoking

C   Risk of death from lung cancer is not reduced by giving up smoking

D   There is a 20–40 year lag before changed habits alter the incidence of lung cancer

E   Risk of developing oesophageal cancer is as great for pipe and cigar smokers as it is for cigarette smokers

10.15 **Smoking is a risk factor for**

A   coronary heart disease

B   failure of coronary artery bypass grafts

C   chronic obstructive lung disease

D   death from aneurysm of the aorta

E   the unborn child

10.16 The following statements about stopping smoking are correct:

A It is generally easy to stop
B Ex-smoker status is a stable state
C There are no differences between women and men in stopping and staying stopped
D Short-term use of an anxiolytic sedative may be beneficial
E Nicotine transdermal patches may cause nightmares

10.17 The following statements about passive smoking are correct:

A Passive smoking means breathing environmental air contaminated by smoke generated by oneself
B Mainstream and sidestream cigarette smoke have the same composition
C Concentrations of carbon monoxide in the air at a party can be × 4 those in smoke-free air
D The balance of evidence favours a small causal effect for lung cancer
E Children whose parents smoke are more prone to respiratory illness than are those of nonsmoking parents

10.18 Ethyl alcohol (alcohol) characteristically causes

A loss of finer grades of judgement and attention even at low doses
B loss of power to control mood
C increase in physical efficiency
D peripheral vasoconstriction
E increased secretion of antidiuretic hormone

10.19 The following statements about alcohol are correct:

A Orientals tend to more tolerant of alcohol than Caucasians

B After an initial increase in blood glucose alcohol causes hypoglycaemia which can be severe

C Vomiting is entirely due to a direct gastric irritant action

D In acute overdose inhalation of vomit is a common cause of death

E A pregnant woman who will not abstain should not exceed 1–2 units per week

10.20 Dependence on and chronic consumption of alcohol are characterised by

A slight emotional dependence

B trivial physical dependence

C hypertension

D absence of tolerance

E deficiency of B group vitamins

10.21 The following statements about alcohol are correct:

A Alcohol acts in the manner of general inhalation anaesthetics

B Food, especially milk, delays absorption

C Habitual drinkers metabolise alcohol less rapidly than non-habitual drinkers

D There are no physical benefits to long-term consumption of alcohol

E Alcohol is subject to saturation or zero-order kinetics

10.22 The following statements about consumption of alcoholic beverages are correct:

A Dehydration due to diuresis is a common cause of 'hangover'
B Alcohol does not pass into breast milk
C Heavy drinkers develop hepatic cirrhosis at a rate of about 2% per annum
D There is no biochemical marker for heavy alcohol consumption
E A standard bottle of spirits (e.g. gin, whisky) contains more alcohol than an average person can metabolise in 24 hours

10.23 Chronic alcohol dependence is characterised by

A psychotic states
B deficiency of vitamin K-dependent clotting factors
C increased high density lipoprotein concentrations
D peripheral neuropathy
E cardiomyopathy

10.24 Acute overdose of alcohol can lead to

A excited and violent behaviour which is best controlled by a barbiturate given intramuscularly
B an episode of acute hepatitis
C fall in serum transaminase
D hypothermia
E hyperuricaemia and acute gout

10.25 Alcohol (ethanol)

A causes nystagmus
B causes increased vigilance at low doses
C increases visual acuity
D induces overconfidence
E reduces reaction time

10.26 The following statement about psychodysleptics and hallucinogens (lysergide or LSD, mescaline etc.) are correct:

A They have no proved therapeutic use
B Their actions cannot be described as precisely as is possible for most other drugs since their effects are highly conditioned by the subject's frame of mind, personality and environment
C They do not cause psychotic reactions
D Physical dependence is characteristic
E 'Bad trips' may be treated with diazepam

10.27 When cannabis is taken

A tolerance does not occur
B visual sensations become more vivid
C cannabinoids are taken up in body fat and slowly released
D recent memory is impaired
E psychotic reactions do not occur

10.28 When cocaine is taken

A in repeated doses, tachyphylaxis (acute tolerance) occurs
B repeatedly as snuff perforation of the nasal septum may occur
C in overdose myocardial infarction may occur
D i.v. the immediate effect is intense euphoria
E hypotension is usual

11 Chemotherapy of infections

11.1 The following drugs are primarily bactericidal:

A Sulphonamides
B Tetracyclines
C Aminoglycosides
D Chloramphenicol
E Rifampicin

11.2 The following statements about the mechanism of action of antimicrobial drugs are correct:

A Penicillin interferes with the bacterial cell wall so that it absorbs water and bursts
B Amphotericin interferes with the cytoplasmic membrane of fungi
C Sulphonamides interfere with the build-up of peptide chains on ribosomes
D Tetracyclines prevent bacteria from synthesising folic acid
E Rifampicin interferes with bacterial nucleic acid metabolism

11.3 The choice of antimicrobial drugs

A may follow automatically from the clinical diagnosis if the causative organism is always the same and is always sensitive to the same drug
B should always be delayed until a positive identification of the infecting organism has been made
C should be based exclusively on in vitro sensitivity tests
D for pyogenic infections should only be altered after a trial of at least one week
E may reasonably be made on the basis of 'best guess'

11.4 Combinations of antimicrobials are useful

A to potentiate drug action, e.g. penicillin plus gentamicin for enterococcal endocarditis
B to delay development of resistance, e.g. in tuberculosis
C where treatment is essential before a diagnosis has been reached
D to reduce the risk of suppression of normal flora
E especially when a bactericidal drug is given with a bacteriostatic drug

11.5 Chemoprophylaxis is justified

A to prevent recurrent attacks of rheumatic fever
B to prevent recurrence of acute glomerulonephritis
C in epidemics of meningococcal meningitis
D to prevent bacterial endocarditis after dental procedures
E to suppress existing infection, e.g. malaria

11.6 Bacterial resistance to antimicrobials can arise

A when naturally sensitive strains are eliminated, allowing naturally resistant organisms to proliferate
B from spontaneous mutation
C when sexual intercourse between cells allows the passage of plasmids
D by passage of bacteriophage from one cell to another
E through drug destroying enzymes produced by bacteria

11.7 Chemoprophylaxis in surgery

A is justified for the insertion of prosthetic joints
B should be given orally
C should be continued for one week after the operation
D is justified following amputation of an ischaemic limb
E should not be used in immunocompromised patients

11.8 **Adverse consequences of antimicrobial drug use may include**

A opportunistic infections by *Clostridium difficile* causing colitis
B opportunistic infection with *Candida albicans*
C masking of infection, e.g. syphilis
D inhibition of alcohol metabolism
E ototoxicity

12 Antibacterial drugs

12.1 Penicillins

A are effective only against multiplying organisms

B are eliminated from the body only by glomerular filtration

C in all forms are resistant to degradation by gastric acid

D are presented as their sodium or potassium salts which may be significant in patients with cardiac or renal disease

E of the aminopenicillin type, e.g. amoxycillin, are indicated for infectious mononucleosis

12.2 Allergic reaction to a penicillin

A may take the form of anaphylactic shock which can be fatal

B in an individual indicates that a cephalosporin may safely be given

C can be relied on to disappear spontaneously with passage of time

D in an individual indicates that another penicillin may safely be given

E may be predicted by testing for specific IgE antibodies in the patient's plasma

12.3 Benzylpenicillin given alone is highly active against

A *Streptococcus pneumoniae* (pneumococcus)

B *Streptococcus pyogenes* (β-haemolytic streptococcus)

C *Staphylococcus pyogenes* (β-lactamase producing)

D *Neisseria meningitidis* (meningococcus)

E *Streptococcus faecalis* causing endocarditis

12.4   The following statements about penicillins are correct:

A   Ampicillin and amoxycillin are destroyed by β-lactamase

B   Flucloxacillin and cloxacillin are resistant to β-lactamase

C   Ticarcillin is particularly effective against *Pseudomonas aeruginosa*

D   Clavulanic acid (a component of co-amoxiclav) has strong antibacterial activity in its own right

E   Piperacillin is inactive against *Pseudomonas aeruginosa*

12.5   Cephalosporins

A   do not have the β-lactam ring in their structure

B   as a rule are excreted unchanged by the kidney

C   should not be used in patients who have had severe or immediate type allergic reactions to penicillin

D   in general have plasma $t_{\frac{1}{2}}$s of less than 3 h

E   may cause thrombocytopenia and neutropenia if administration is continued for longer than 2 weeks

12.6   The following statements about imipenem and vancomycin are correct:

A   Imipenem has a narrow spectrum of antibacterial activity

B   Imipenem is inactivated by metabolism in the kidney

C   Vancomycin is effective by the oral route to treat systemic infections

D   Vancomycin is effective against *Clostridium difficile*

E   Vancomycin may usefully be combined with an aminoglycoside to treat streptococcal endocarditis

12.7   Aminoglycosides

A   are in general inactivated by metabolism in the liver

B   are in general active against aerobic Gram-negative organisms

C   are unsuitable to use in regimens to sterilise the bowel

D   may cause nephrotoxicity

E   such as neomycin used topically may be absorbed sufficiently to cause ototoxicity

12.8 Sulphonamides

A act by preventing bacterial synthesis of folic acid
B are more active after metabolism to the acetylated form
C are suitable for topical use
D may cause crystalluria
E may cause the Stevens–Johnson syndrome

12.9 The following statements about co-trimoxazole and trimethoprim are correct:

A Co-trimoxazole is the treatment of choice for pneumonia due to *Pneumocystis carinii*
B Co-trimoxazole is used for the prevention and treatment of toxoplasmosis
C Trimethoprim is effective against *Pseudomonas aeruginosa*
D Trimethoprim is excreted largely unchanged in the urine
E Co-trimoxazole is a combination of trimethoprim and clavulanic acid

12.10 A member of the tetracycline class of antibiotic

A is better absorbed from the intestinal tract if taken with dairy products
B is as a rule excreted unchanged in the urine
C such as demeclocycline may be used to treat hyponatraemia due to the syndrome of inappropriate antidiuretic hormone secretion
D is a treatment of choice for psittacosis
E is a treatment of choice for mycoplasma pneumonia

12.11 Tetracyclines can cause

A liver damage, especially in pregnancy
B decreased sensitivity to dental caries
C photosensitisation
D opportunistic infection with yeasts and moulds
E serious growth retardation in children treated for chronic respiratory disease

12.12 The following statements about antimicrobial drugs are correct:

A Erythromycin is the drug of choice for Legionnaires' disease

B Erythromycin estolate can cause cholestatic hepatitis

C Metronidazole is effective for trichomoniasis of the urogenital tract

D Metronidazole is ineffective for infection with anaerobic organisms

E Metronidazole use may cause peripheral neuritis

12.13 The following statements about antimicrobial drugs are correct:

A Chloramphenicol is inactivated slowly by the neonate

B Chloramphenicol is effective treatment for infection with *Haemophilus influenzae*

C Aplastic anaemia due to chloramphenicol may be either an allergy or a dose-related response

D Clarithromycin is ineffective treatment for atypical pneumonia

E Sodium fusidate is effective treatment for staphylococcal osteomyelitis

12.14 The following statements about antimicrobial drugs are correct:

A Ciprofloxacin impairs the metabolism of theophylline to a clinically significant degree

B Acrosoxacin is an alternative for penicillin in gonorrhoea

C Vancomycin plus an aminoglycoside is effective treatment for streptococcal endocarditis in patients who are allergic to benzylpenicillin

D Quinolone antimicrobials may cause rupture of the Achilles tendon

E Mupirocin is much more effective in the treatment of folliculitis and impetigo if given systemically rather than topically

13 Chemotherapy of bacterial infections

13.1   In a case of septicaemia

A   treatment is so urgent that it should be started before taking blood cultures

B   in neonates is usually due to streptococci or coliforms

C   *Staphylococcus aureus* is a likely cause where there is an abscess

D   antimicrobials should be given orally

E   due to urinary tract infection, *Pseudomonas aeruginosa* may be the pathogen

13.2   The following statements are correct:

A   *Haemophilus influenzae* is not a likely cause of infection of the auditory canal in children

B   Middle ear infection may be caused by *Moraxella catarrhalis*

C   In sinusitis, antimicrobials have dispensed with the need to promote normal drainage

D   A bulging inflamed eardrum may demand treatment by myringotomy

E   In sinusitis, *Streptococcus pneumoniae* is a common pathogen

13.3 In throat infections

A due to *Streptococcus pyogenes* (Group A), benzylpenicillin is frequently ineffective

B severe sporadic or epidemic sore throat is likely to be streptococcal

C chemoprophylaxis should be continued for life after a second attack of rheumatic fever

D due to *Bordetella pertussis* (whooping cough), erythromycin is recommended at the catarrhal stage

E due to diphtheria, there is no longer any need for antitoxin, provided that erythromycin is used

13.4 In the treatment of bronchitis

A acute infection responds well to amoxycillin

B suppressive chemotherapy for chronic infection is generally needed only during the colder months in temperate regions

C trimethoprim is an appropriate drug

D *Klebsiella pneumoniae* should be considered a common pathogen

E if an exacerbation lasts for more than 10 days, there is a need for clinical reassessment

13.5 The following statements about pneumonia are correct:

A A cephalosporin is preferable to benzylpenicillin for all patients with lobar pneumonia

B Atypical pneumonia due to *Mycoplasma pneumoniae* is best treated with amoxycillin

C Initial therapy for nosocomial (hospital acquired) pneumonia may reasonably be ciprofloxacin

D *Pneumocystis carinii* pneumonia in a patient suffering from AIDS is treated by co-trimoxazole

E Legionnaires' disease responds to benzylpenicillin

13.6 In infective endocarditis

A treatment should not be delayed once blood cultures have been taken, even if the organism has not been identified

B bacteriostatic antimicrobials are preferred for therapy

C in intravenous drug abusers, *Staphylococcus aureus* is the commonest pathogen

D antimicrobial therapy for 10 days is sufficient

E treatment with continuous intravenous infusion of antimicrobials is preferred

13.7 With regard to the prophylaxis of infective endocarditis in patients who are at risk

A an antimicrobial should be administered for two days prior to a dental or surgical procedure

B patients with prosthetic valves who are undergoing general anaesthesia should receive amoxycillin and gentamicin

C antibiotic cover is obligatory for endoscopic procedures

D all oral drugs should be taken under supervision

E patients undergoing tonsillectomy who are allergic to penicillin require intravenous vancomycin and gentamicin

13.8 In the management of meningitis

A rifampicin by mouth should be given to close personal contacts of those who have the infection

B due to *Haemophilus influenzae* the patient is likely to respond to benzylpenicillin

C of meningococcal origin, benzylpenicillin is the drug of choice

D due to *Streptococcus pneumoniae*, antimicrobial therapy should continue for 10 days after the patient has become afebrile

E due to *Mycobacterium tuberculosis*, isoniazid is of little value because of its failure to penetrate well into the CSF

13.9 The following statements about intestinal infections are correct:

A Amoxycillin in high dose by mouth for 3 months may be necessary to eradicate *Salmonella typhi* from carriers

B Even quite mild shigellosis demands treatment with co-trimoxazole

C *Campylobacter jejuni* infection should be treated with erythromycin

D In cholera the most important aim of treatment remains rehydration and the maintenance of fluid balance

E A quinolone is the preferred treatment for infection with *Escherichia coli*

13.10 In the treatment of urinary tract infections

A gentamicin is preferred to amoxicillin for asymptomatic infection in pregnancy

B cefotaxime i.v. is a suitable treatment when the upper urinary tract is involved

C nitrofurantoin is a suitable drug for acute infections

D nalidixic acid is suitable for prevention

E chemoprophylaxis may prevent subclinical renal damage in young girls with asymptomatic bacteriuria

13.11 In the treatment of infections of the genital tract

A *Treponema pallidum* never becomes resistant to penicillin

B a tetracycline in high dose may be needed for pharyngeal gonorrhoea

C nonspecific vaginitis responds well to metronidazole

D nongonococcal urethritis does not respond to tetracycline

E the Herxheimer reaction is probably caused by cytokine release

13.12 In eye infections

A superficial infection with *Staphylococcus aureus* responds to fusidic acid administered topically

B a corticosteroid administered topically as sole therapy is useful in herpes simplex keratitis

C gentamicin drops are suitable for superficial infection with *Pseudomonas aeruginosa*

D due to chlamydia, a tetracycline is effective

E local antibacterial chemoprophylaxis is useful to prevent secondary invasion in viral conjunctivitis

13.13 The following statements about antituberculosis treatment are correct:

A A combination of isoniazid, pyrazinamide and rifampicin is the cornerstone of short-course chemotherapy regimens

B Noncompliance is the chief reason for failure of chemotherapy

C Isoniazid is highly effective against actively multiplying organisms

D Rifampicin and pyrazinamide are most efficacious against semidormant bacilli

E Persons known to be in contact with the disease and who develop a positive tuberculin reaction should always receive antituberculosis chemotherapy

13.14 Isoniazid

A has little or no activity against bacteria other than *Mycobacterium tuberculosis*

B acts as efficiently in genetic fast acetylators as in slow acetylators in standard oral doses

C may cause severe hepatitis

D may cause peripheral neuropathy which is preventable with pyridoxine

E may interfere with antiepilepsy therapy

13.15 Rifampicin

A has a bactericidal action against tubercle bacilli
B is effective in leprosy
C given intermittently may provoke an influenza-like syndrome
D may safely be given to a woman receiving an oral contraceptive
E causes an orange discolouration in soft contact lenses

13.16 Adverse effects of

A ethambutol include monocular retrobulbar neuritis
B pyrazinamide include arthralgia associated with a raised plasma uric acid
C rifampicin on the liver, with rise in plasma bilirubin and transaminase enzymes, are an absolute indication for stopping the drug
D thiacetazone includes erythema multiforme
E dapsone include haemolytic anaemia

13.17 The following statements are correct:

A Penicillin may be used to prevent gas gangrene after mid-thigh amputations
B Neomycin applied to burned surfaces may be absorbed in amounts sufficient to cause ototoxicity
C Metronidazole is the treatment of choice for staphylococcal osteomyelitis
D Benzylpenicillin is the treatment of choice for leptospirosis
E *Borrelia burgdorferi* (the cause of Lyme disease) is sensitive to amoxycillin

14 Viral, fungal, protozoal and helminthic infections

14.1   Aciclovir

A   acts by inhibiting viral DNA synthesis
B   is absorbed from the gut in amounts sufficient to treat viral encephalitis
C   is effective as an ointment for ocular herpes simplex keratitis
D   is ineffective against *Varicella-zoster* virus
E   toxicity severely limits its use

14.2   In the chemotherapy of acquired immuno deficiency syndrome (AIDS)

A   zidovudine is a reverse transcriptase inhibitor
B   zidovudine may cause a toxic myopathy
C   the long intracellular residence of didanosine is an advantage
D   indinavir acts by protease inhibition
E   antivirus drugs are best used singly rather than in combination

14.3   In the treatment of

A   influenza A, amantadine is effective
B   sight-threatening cytomegalovirus infection, ganciclovir is used
C   respiratory syncytial virus infection, tribavirin is effective as an aerosol
D   hairy cell leukaemia, interferon alfa is effective
E   hepatitis B and C, interferon alfa is ineffective

14.4   In the chemotherapy of fungal infections

A   lipid-associated formulations of amphotericin are associated with reduced toxicity

B   amphotericin remains the drug of choice for most systemic infections

C   ketoconazole impairs testosterone synthesis to a clinically significant degree

D   griseofulvin acts not by killing fungus but by preventing infection of new keratin

E   fluconazole may safely be given to pregnant women

14.5   The following statements about the treatment of an acute attack of malaria are correct:

A   Quinine no longer has a significant role to play

B   Chloroquine will eradicate hepatic parasites

C   A course of pyrimethamine plus sulfadoxine (Fansidar) reduces the rate of relapse

D   Mefloquine may be used for falciparum malaria

E   Primaquine should be given for infection with *Plasmodium malariae*

14.6   The following statements about the prevention of malaria by drugs in visitors to an endemic area are correct:

A   A significant reason for beginning prophylaxis before travel is to reveal adverse effects in advance

B   Preventive efficacy depends on continuing the drug for four weeks after leaving the endemic area

C   Mefloquine may safely be given to a pregnant woman

D   Proguanil may be given to a pregnant woman provided it is accompanied by folic acid

E   The partially immune as a rule should not take a drug prophylactically

14.7   The following statements about chloroquine are correct:

   A   Resistance to chloroquine is uncommon
   B   Chloroquine acts against the plasmodium in its hepatic
       cycle
   C   Diazepam and adrenaline are effective against
       chloroquine in overdose
   D   Chloroquine may cause visual field defects
   E   Pruritus with chloroquine is particularly severe in Africans

**14.8   The following statements about antimalarial drugs are
         correct:**

   A   Primaquine is liable to cause haemolysis in persons with
       glucose-6-phosphate dehydrogenase deficiency
   B   Halofantrine prolongs the cardiac QT interval and may
       predispose to severe dysrhythmia
   C   Mefloquine is contraindicated in airline pilots
   D   Primaquine is used to eliminate the hepatic forms of
       Plasmodium vivax and *Plasmodium ovale*
   E   Quinine overdose may cause blindness

14.9   In amoebiasis

   A   metronidazole is the agent of first choice for symptomatic
       tissue-invading disease
   B   dehydroemetine may cause cardiotoxicity
   C   diloxanide is useful in eradicating the cystic forms from
       the bowel lumen
   D   tetracycline has a part to play in the treatment of severe
       cases with extensive ulceration
   E   treatment with tissue amoebicides is sufficient to
       eradicate bowel lumen amoebiasis

14.10 The following statements about protozoal and helminthic infections are correct:

A Suramin is particularly useful in the treatment of African trypanosomiasis with CNS involvement

B Chronic infection with *Giardia lamblia* responds to metronidazole

C Levamisole acts by paralysing the musculature of sensitive nematodes

D Ivermectin is effective treatment for onchocerciasis (river blindness)

E Diethylcarbamazine is used to treat filariasis

15 Inflammation, arthritis and nonsteroidal anti-inflammatory drugs (NSAIDs)

15.1   The following statements about prostaglandins and leukotrienes are correct:

A   Arachidonic acid is metabolised to form prostaglandins and leukotrienes

B   NSAIDs act by inhibiting prostaglandin G/H synthase

C   Cyclo-oxygenase-1 (COX-1) is noninducible and present in many tissues

D   Cyclo-oxygenase-2 (COX-2) is induced by cytokines at sites of inflammation

E   Actions of leukotrienes include bronchoconstriction

15.2   Nonsteroidal anti-inflammatory drugs

A   cause sodium retention and oedema

B   may be used to attempt closure of a patent ductus arteriosus

C   reduce fever

D   can cause asthma

E   can protect against vascular thrombosis

15.3   Paracetamol taken in acute overdose

A   characteristically causes immediate symptoms

B   is especially dangerous in malnourished patients

C   may be rendered non-toxic by acetylcysteine i.v.

D   is less toxic in enzyme-induced patients

E   may damage the kidneys

15.4 **The following statements about nonsteroidal anti-inflammatory drugs are correct:**

A   Ibuprofen is less likely than aspirin to cause adverse effects in the gastrointestinal tract
B   Mefenamic acid may cause nonoliguric renal failure in the elderly
C   Indomethacin may cause headache
D   Piroxicam may be used topically on the skin for soft tissue trauma
E   Diclofenac is effective for relief of renal colic

15.5 **The following statements about aspirin and salicylates are correct:**

A   Aspirin has a $t_{\frac{1}{2}}$ of 5 hours
B   Salicylate has a $t_{\frac{1}{2}}$ of 15 minutes
C   Aspirin is more toxic to the stomach if taken with sodium bicarbonate
D   Aspirin may cause asthma
E   Aspirin reduces blood platelet adhesiveness

15.6 **Salicylates, including aspirin,**

A   cause respiratory alkalosis in acute overdose
B   stimulate the respiratory centre
C   are metabolised according to zero-order kinetics at high therapeutic doses
D   cause urate retention in ordinary therapeutic dose
E   cause tinnitus in overdose

15.7 Aspirin

A when taken long term causes loss of about 5 ml of blood per day from the gastrointestinal tract in most people

B taking is epidemiologically related to the development of Reye's syndrome

C may cause gastrointestinal haemorrhage after a single dose

D when enteric-coated, causes less gastrointestinal bleeding

E taken as a rapidly dispersible tablet swallowed as a liquid is more likely to be associated with gastric bleeding

15.8 Aspirin poisoning

A is benefited by urinary acidification

B is benefited by activated charcoal in repeated doses

C may cause severe metabolic acidosis especially in children under 4 years

D should be regarded as severe if the plasma salicylate exceeds 750 mg/l

E even if severe will not respond to haemodialysis

15.9 In the treatment of rheumatoid arthritis

A a propionic acid derivative is a reasonable first choice for mild disease

B regular measurements of plasma salicylate are mandatory if aspirin is used

C slow-acting antirheumatic drugs should be introduced early once the diagnosis of rheumatoid arthritis is established

D sulphasalazine is the most toxic of the slow-acting antirheumatic drugs

E adverse effects of gold may be treated with a chelating agent

15.10 In the treatment of rheumatoid arthritis

A hydroxychloroquine gives benefit within 4 days
B if gold fails to achieve a response after 4 months another drug should be used
C methylprednisolone 1 g monthly for 1–3 months may be given to relieve exacerbations of the disease
D prednisolone 7.5 mg/day is effective for rheumatoid lung
E intra-articular injections of corticosteroid into a single joint should not exceed 3 per year

15.11 The following statements about hyperuricaemia and gout are correct:

A Patients with gouty tophi have a urate pool that is 15–26 times normal
B Hyperuricaemia may result from treatment of a myeloproliferative disorder
C Colchicine relieves pain and inflammation of gout in a few hours
D Probenecid is a useful analgesic for gout
E Initiating treatment with allopurinol may precipitate an attack of acute gout

15.12 In the treatment of gout

A allopurinol acts as a uricosuric
B in an acute attack prednisolone 40 mg/day may be used if nonsteroidal anti-inflammatory drugs fail to give relief in a few hours
C allopurinol alone will provide useful relief from an acute attack
D a salicylate should be combined with a uricosuric
E a diuretic may cause relapse

16 Drugs and the skin

16.1   When a drug is applied to the skin

A   absorption is greater if an occlusive dressing is used
B   some presystemic (first-pass) metabolism may occur in the epidermis and dermis
C   it is of little importance what vehicle is used
D   its pharmacokinetics are influenced by the state of the keratin layer
E   absorption from the palm of the hand is high relative to other areas

16.2   Lotions

A   are contraindicated in acutely inflamed lesions
B   are less useful if there is much exudation
C   exert their soothing effect through the evaporation of water
D   after evaporation, may produce excessive drying of the skin
E   applied over large areas can reduce body temperature dangerously in old people

16.3   The following statements about skin creams are correct:

A   An oil-in-water cream mixes with serous discharges
B   Water-in-oil creams are more easy to spread than ointments
C   Pastes are used to protect circumscribed lesions
D   Silicone sprays are useful in the prevention and treatment of pressure sores
E   Masking creams are used mostly to protect against sunburn

16.4 In the therapy of skin disease

A nonemulsifying preparations such as paraffin ointment are particularly useful to deliver active agents on hairy areas

B pastes are ointments containing insoluble powders

C Zinc Starch and Talc Dusting-powder is likely to increase friction between skin surfaces

D water-soluble ointments are unsuitable as vehicles for the passage of drugs into the skin

E collodions are used to hold a medicament in contact with the skin

16.5 Pruritus

A is dependent on both central and peripheral mechanisms

B if generalised may respond to a histamine H_2-receptor blocker taken systemically

C in partial obstructive jaundice may be treated with cholestyramine by mouth

D responds to long-term use of a local anaesthetic applied topically

E if generalised may be treated with topical hydrocortisone

16.6 When an adrenocorticosteroid preparation is used in skin disease

A systemic treatment should only be given in a serious condition such as pemphigus

B topical application does not allow sufficient absorption to cause systemic toxicity

C abrupt withdrawal does not exacerbate disease

D a potent fluorinated steroid is first choice for facial conditions

E skin atrophy and striae may follow local application

16.7 **Adrenal steroids have a place in the treatment of**

A alopecia areata
B severe exfoliative dermatitis
C herpes simplex
D rosacea
E dermatitis herpetiformis

16.8 **Sunscreens**

A of the absorbent type are generally more effective against ultraviolet radiation B (UVB)
B of the reflective type consist of organic chemicals
C ought in general to provide for protection against UVC
D are rated for their performance by the sun protective factor (SPF)
E are ineffective against drug-induced photosensitivity

16.9 **Photosensitivity**

A may be produced by amiodarone
B sometimes follows the use of shaving lotions and sunscreens containing 6-methylcoumarin
C may be induced with psoralens
D in the form of polymorphic light eruptions can be prevented by the short-term use of chloroquine
E of the photoallergy type may persist for years after the causal drug has been discontinued

16.10 **Drugs given systemically may cause**

A erythema multiforme
B erythema nodosum
C exfoliative dermatitis
D urticaria and angioedema
E hair loss

16.11 Dermal adverse reactions

A to systemically administered drugs are commonly erythematous

B due to local contact are nearly always urticarial

C are usually of the same kind in all patients who take the offending drug

D manifest as fixed eruptions may reasonably be diagnosed by readministration of a suspect drug

E due to drugs usually occur during the first two weeks of therapy

16.12 Psoriasis

A can be rationally treated with oestrogen-containing creams

B is associated with increased numbers of horn cells containing abnormal keratin

C of the scalp is often treated by tar preparations

D can sometimes be helped by psoralens

E in a woman of child-bearing potential may be treated with acitretin without risk of teratogenicity

16.13 In the treatment of acne

A keratolytic agents are used to unblock pilosebaceous ducts

B tretinoin should not be used in sunny weather

C tetracycline suppresses the bacterial lipolysis of sebum

D there is no place for an antiandrogen such as cyproterone

E a topical corticosteroid is valuable

16.14 In the treatment of skin infections

A due to bacteria, mupirocin is suitable for topical use

B neomycin ointment may be absorbed in sufficient quantity to cause deafness if used on large areas

C cellulitis should be treated with a topically-administered antimicrobial drug

D use of fusidic acid topically is best confined to hospitals

E topical malathion is used for pediculosis

16.15 The following statements are correct:

A Alopecia areata is often self-limiting
B Dapsone is effective for dermatitis herpetiformis
C Cyproterone plus ethinyloestradiol may be used to treat severe hirsutism in women
D Warts often disappear spontaneously
E Permethrin dermal cream is effective for scabies

17 Pain and analgesics

17.1 **The following statements about pain and analgesics are correct:**

A Pain is the commonest symptom that takes a patient to a doctor

B Pain is defined as an unpleasant sensory, but not emotional, experience that occurs only in association with actual tissue damage

C All drugs that relieve pain should be classed as analgesics

D Non-narcotic drugs relieve pain by central action

E Nonanalgesic, e.g. psychotropic, drugs can be useful adjuvants alongside analgesics

17.2 **Pain is a complex phenomenon composed of a variable mix of**

A nociceptive input

B input from other receptors

C anxiety, fear

D depression

E synthesis and release of local tissue hormones, e.g. prostaglandins, which cause inflammation and sensitise nerve endings that mediate pain

17.3 The following statements about pain are correct:

A Pain is a consequence of the activation of specific pain receptors in the affected tissue
B Acute and chronic pain are treated similarly
C Tissue injury always gives rise to pain
D Anxiety can intensify pain
E Depression makes a major contribution to 'suffering'

17.4 The following statements about pain are correct:

A Analgesia is associated with μ and κ opioid receptors
B Dysphoria is associated with σ opioid receptors
C Naloxone competitively opposes administered opioids
D Naloxone does not cause spontaneous pain, but can make existing pain worse
E Nonsteroidal anti-inflammatory drugs benefit pain by preventing prostaglandin synthesis

17.5 The following statements about acute and chronic pain are correct:

A Acute pain is transmitted by fast conducting A-delta nerve fibres
B In chronic pain antidepressant drugs can often be useful
C In chronic pain it is best to inject analgesics
D In chronic pain an analgesic with sedative action is preferred
E In acute pain, morphine is useful because of both antinociceptive and antianxiety effects

17.6 The following statements about testing of analgesic drugs are correct:

A Placebos give relief in about 3% of (healthy or nonpatient) volunteers undergoing experimental studies of pain
B Emotional response to pain can largely be ignored in healthy volunteer experiments
C Double-blind technique is unnecessary
D Animal experiments are valueless
E The gender of the experimenter/observer may influence the responses of the trial subjects

17.7 **The following statements about the choice of analgesics are correct:**

A Analgesia for mild pain is best provided by paracetamol or aspirin

B Analgesia for moderate pain is best provided by a low-efficacy opioid combined if necessary with a nonsteroidal anti-inflammatory drug

C Severe pain requires a high efficacy opioid combined with a low-efficacy opioid

D Overwhelming acute pain responds to a high-efficacy opioid plus a psychotropic drug, e.g. chlorpromazine

E The inclusion of caffeine in fixed-ratio analgesic combinations has no scientific basis

17.8 **Pain**

A from visceral smooth muscle responds best to aspirin

B from spasm of striated muscle should first be treated with an opioid

C of thalamic origin may respond to chlorpromazine

D of trigeminal neuralgia should in the first instance be treated with pentazocine

E of postherpetic neuralgia may be relieved by transcutaneous nerve stimulation

17.9 **In a migraine attack**

A the nondispersible form of aspirin is preferred to the dispersible form

B use of the enteral form of ergotamine should not exceed 6 mg

C serotonergic neurons may be involved in its initiation

D the pain is due to extracerebral vasoconstriction

E sumatriptan acts by vasoconstriction via stimulating '5-HT$_1$-like' receptors

17.10 Drugs that are useful in an acute attack of migraine include

A paracetamol
B metoclopramide
C a benzodiazepine
D pethidine
E cyclizine

17.11 Ergotamine

A is valuable for preventing migraine
B in overdose can cause gangrene of the extremities by its α-adrenoceptor agonist action
C is safe to use in pregnancy
D may be given by inhalation
E should not be used within 6 h of the last dose of sumatriptan

17.12 Drugs that may be useful in prevention of recurrent migraine include

A aspirin
B propranolol
C verapamil
D pizotifen
E methysergide

17.13 The following statements regarding care of the terminally ill are correct:

A Symptom control is all-important to provide optimal quality of life
B Drugs play only a minor role in symptom control
C Initial drowsiness with morphine tends to diminish with passage of time
D Tricyclic antidepressants have a morphine-sparing effect
E Amphetamine may be used to elevate mood

17.14 In the patient terminally ill with cancer

A dependence on regularly administered opioids becomes a serious problem

B acquired tolerance to regularly administered opioids should be anticipated

C anorexia may be helped by prednisolone

D headache due to raised intracranial pressure responds to dexamethasone

E and in continuous pain, the interval between doses of analgesics should be short enough to prevent pain recurring

17.15 The following statements about opioid analgesics are correct:

A Pure morphine-like opioid agonists in general act on μ- and κ-receptors

B Naltrexone is a pure competitive opioid receptor antagonist

C Opioid drugs may be an agonist to one class of opioid receptor and an antagonist at another

D A single opioid may exert dual agonist/antagonist effect on a single receptor according to circumstances

E Codeine, a weak (low efficacy) agonist, potentiates the therapeutic effect of morphine (high efficacy)

17.16 Morphine

A stimulates some functions of the central nervous system

B depresses some functions of the central nervous system

C dilates the biliary tract

D dilates resistance (arterioles) and capacitance (veins) vessels

E may produce dysphoria

17.17 Morphine can cause

A histamine release

B vomiting

C cough suppression

D antidiuresis

E miosis

17.18 Morphine should if possible be avoided in patients with

A pancreatitis
B asthma
C respiratory depression
D acute left ventricular failure
E constipation

17.19 Morphine may safely be given

A subcutaneously to shocked patients
B to patients with hepatic failure
C together with a tricyclic antidepressant
D together with a monoamine oxidase inhibitor
E to a patient with (untreated) severe hypothyroidism

17.20 Morphine and heroin dependence

A is more disabling socially and physically than is opium dependence
B should be treated by abrupt withdrawal of the drug
C is acceptable in the management of chronic pain in the terminally ill
D can commence within 24 hours if the drug is given 4-hourly
E can occur in infants born to addicted mothers

17.21 Codeine

A is as effective an analgesic as morphine
B does not constipate
C is a useful antitussive
D causes excitement in large doses
E is partly metabolised into morphine in the body

17.22 Pethidine

A has higher therapeutic efficacy than does morphine
B is preferred above codeine for cough suppression
C constipates
D is used in labour in preference to morphine
E has strong hypnotic effect

17.23 Methadone

A has a much longer duration of action than that of morphine and pethidine
B dependence is less severe than is morphine dependence
C is widely used (orally) to help wean addicts from injected heroin
D blocks the acute effects of injected heroin
E is useful for severe cough

17.24 Heroin (diamorphine)

A is unsuitable for administration by continuous s.c. infusion
B provides more rapid relief of pain than morphine
C is more potent (weight for weight) than morphine
D is metabolised in the body to morphine and to 6-acetylmorphine
E is used for very severe cough

17.25 The following statements about opioids are correct:

A Pentazocine and buprenorphine are partial opioid agonists
B Pentazocine may induce a withdrawal syndrome in opioid (heroin, morphine) dependent subjects
C Partial agonist opioids are free from the classic opioid adverse effects
D Neither pentazocine nor buprenorphine induces dependence
E Etorphine (formulated for large animal immobilisation) has killed humans when spread in the skin

17.26 Naloxone

A is a noncompetitive opioid antagonist
B is effective treatment for opioid overdose
C is longer-acting than is morphine
D only partially antagonises buprenorphine in overdose
E does not induce an acute withdrawal syndrome in heroin addicts

18 Sleep and anxiety

18.1 **The following statements about sleep are correct:**

A Normal sleep is an active circadian depression of consciousness

B The kinds of sleep may be characterised by eye movement patterns or electroencephalographic patterns

C About 30% of adults have difficulty in sleeping

D Normal sleep patterns are resumed immediately on withdrawal of a hypnotic after a period of continuous use

E All hypnotics can induce dependence

18.2 **The following statements about hypnotics are correct:**

A If a patient does not feel a hangover after a hypnotic he can count on his psychomotor performance being normal

B Hypnotics are best taken one hour before going to bed

C After a long period of continuous use a hypnotic should be withdrawn slowly over weeks

D Long-term use of a hypnotic is appropriate for persistent insomnia

E The elderly are tolerant of hypnotics

18.3 In treating insomnia

A prescription of a hypnotic is not justified to help a patient through a sudden distressing situation, e.g., bereavement, as it is just this sort of use that carries risk of dependence

B alcohol, while helping people to get to sleep, can cause early morning waking

C it is important to make a detailed enquiry into its cause and pattern

D it should be remembered that sleep requirement becomes less with increasing age

E benzodiazepines are the first choice as hypnotics

18.4 The following statements about anxiety are correct:

A Anxiety is always harmful

B Anxiety does not always have an environmental or life-situational cause

C Nondrug therapy is a waste of time

D A β-adrenoceptor blocker may give benefit

E Long-term use of a benzodiazepine is desirable to ensure there is no relapse of anxiety

18.5 In the treatment of anxiety

A psychic symptoms respond particularly well to β-adrenoceptor blocking drugs

B somatic symptoms should be treated with an α-adrenoceptor blocking drug

C in an alcoholic patient, chlormethiazole is appropriate

D benzodiazepines with a short $t_{\frac{1}{2}}$ are preferred in chronic cases

E with benzodiazepines, some tolerance can generally be expected to develop

18.6 Benzodiazepines

A are appropriate treatment for panic attacks
B only rarely induce dependence
C are without efficacy in epilepsy
D in overdose are particularly liable to cause respiratory depression
E can cause paradoxical excitement and aggression

18.7 Benzodiazepines

A reduce the activity of a central neurotransmitter, GABA (gamma-aminobutyric acid)
B cause anterograde amnesia
C are used as sedatives for endoscopy
D do not sedate sufficiently to render car driving inadvisable
E given to a mother in labour may depress suckling in the new-born infant

18.8 Benzodiazepines

A alter sleep pattern more than do other hypnotics
B are potent inducers of hepatic drug metabolising enzymes
C are safer if taken in overdose than are other hypnotics
D all have pharmacologically active metabolites
E having a long $t_{\frac{1}{2}}$ are best for repeated use in insomnia

18.9 The following statements are correct:

A Cimetidine increases the plasma concentration of diazepam
B Flumazenil selectively reverses the effects of benzodiazepines
C Alprazolam has an antidepressant as well as a sedative action
D Lorazepam is particularly liable to cause dependence
E Benzodiazepines in large dose may induce sexual fantasies in women

18.10 **The following statements about hypnotics and sedatives are correct:**

A Zopiclone has a pronounced hangover effect
B Paraldehyde dissolves plastic syringes
C Chloral hydrate has a pleasant taste
D Zolpidem has a longer $t_{\frac{1}{2}}$ than most benzodiazepines
E Chlormethiazole is used during withdrawal from chronic alcohol abuse

18.11 **Barbiturates**

A have a low therapeutic index
B in overdose may cause coma lasting for days
C are potent inducers of hepatic drug metabolising enzymes
D cause only mild physical dependence
E have been popular drugs of social abuse

19 Drugs and mental disorder

19.1 Psychotropic drugs

A act by modifying chemotransmitter systems in the nervous system
B can be evaluated for therapeutic efficacy by rating scales
C which act in the reticular activating system, particularly influence arousal
D which act in the limbic system, particularly influence affect or emotion
E which act in the hypothalamus, particularly influence the autonomic system

19.2 Schizophrenic states

A are particularly associated with dopaminergic activity in the brain
B are benefited by drugs that block dopamine D_2-receptors
C are benefited by the phenothiazine group of neuroleptics
D manifesting themselves with negative symptoms, e.g. apathy, respond particularly well to drug therapy
E manifesting themselves with positive symptoms, e.g. delusions, respond particularly poorly to drug therapy

19.3 The following statements about adverse effects of neuroleptic drugs are correct:

A Extrapyramidal motor effects of drugs that block dopamine receptors, e.g. phenothiazines, can be alleviated by antimuscarinic drugs, e.g. benztropine

B Phenothiazines that also have antimuscarinic actions are more likely to cause extrapyramidal disorders

C Akathisia due to dopamine-receptor blockers responds to β-blockade

D When tardive dyskinesia develops, it is usually after 2–5 years exposure to a dopamine-receptor blocker

E Tetrabenazine may benefit tardive dyskinesia

19.4 Depressive states

A are particularly associated with cholinergic activity in the brain

B are benefited by drugs that block adrenoceptors in the brain

C respond to drugs after 7–14 days

D respond to electroconvulsive therapy more slowly than to drugs

E may respond to inhibition of serotonin re-uptake

19.5 The following statements about mania and manic depressive disorder are correct:

A Mania may be accompanied by overactivity of catecholamine transmission in the brain

B Lithium takes 2–3 weeks to provide benefit in mania

C Lithium is used to prevent relapse in mania

D Haloperidol is a drug of first choice for acute mania

E Levodopa may cause mania

19.6 **The following statements about the management of depression are correct:**

A Lithium is the most effective drug for the prophylaxis of manic depressive disorder

B Insomnia of depression may respond to an antidepressant alone

C Electroconvulsive (ECT) therapy may benefit depression when a tricyclic antidepressant fails

D Antidepressant drugs can precipitate epilepsy

E Reactive depression with anxiety may be treated with a benzodiazepine alone

19.7 **The following statements are correct:**

A Narcolepsy is worsened by drugs that activate noradrenergic mechanisms

B Children with attention deficit disorder are benefited by dexamphetamine

C Nocturnal enuresis in children can be controlled by a tricyclic antidepressant

D Enhancement of cholinergic function may benefit senile dementias of Alzheimer type

E Excessive sex drive in men may be aggravated by cyproterone

19.8 **Psychotropic drugs may be classified as**

A neuroleptics

B anxiolytic sedatives

C antidepressants

D psychostimulants

E psychodysleptics

19.9 In psychiatry

A environmental factors can be ignored in assessing response to drugs
B dosage of drug can be readily and precisely adjusted according to clinical response
C ideal therapeutic response may occur at intermediate plasma concentrations of some antidepressants
D where therapeutic response is difficult to measure the plasma drug concentration is normally used as a guide
E dose increments should be added at intervals that take into account the half-life of the drug

19.10 Actions of neuroleptics include

A dopamine receptor block
B α-adrenoceptor block
C β-adrenoceptor block
D antimuscarinic effects
E potentiation of cerebral depressants

19.11 Adverse reactions to phenothiazine neuroleptics include

A cholestatic jaundice
B akathisia
C dry mouth
D galactorrhoea
E tardive dyskinesia

19.12 With injected (i.m.) long-acting depot neuroleptics

A patient noncompliance is halved
B defaulters are identifiable
C hepatic first-pass metabolism is enhanced
D extrapyramidal syndromes are common and are treated by an antimuscarinic drug
E severe depression can occur

19.13 The following statements about tricyclic antidepressants are correct:

A Muscarinic adverse effects are common
B Interactions with sympathomimetics and antihypertensives are clinically important
C Use in patients with a history of cardiac disease is safe
D β-adrenoceptor blockade may be of benefit in cases of overdose
E Abuse is a problem

19.14 The following statements about tricyclic antidepressants are correct:

A Imipramine should be given in the evening
B Amitriptyline should be given in the morning
C They may safely be withdrawn abruptly after chronic use
D They may benefit nocturnal enuresis
E They are of use in chronic pain

19.15 Nonselective monoamine oxidase (MAO) inhibitors

A cause decrease in catecholamines and 5-hydroxytryptamine in the central nervous system
B allow increased absorption of monoamines from the gut
C mostly act irreversibly
D potentiate injected sympathomimetics that act directly on adrenoceptors (e.g. adrenaline in local anaesthetic)
E potentiate injected sympathomimetics that act indirectly by causing release of noradrenaline stores

19.16 Patients on treatment with nonselective monoamine oxidase inhibitors are at risk of hypertensive reactions if they consume

A milk
B yoghurt
C soy sauce
D matured cheese
E broad bean pods

19.17 In a hypertensive crisis in a patient taking a monoamine oxidase inhibitor, immediate control of the blood pressure will be achievable with

A propranolol
B methyldopa
C captopril
D nifedipine
E phentolamine

19.18 The following statements about lithium are correct:

A Sustained release formulations are particularly to be avoided
B It is distributed throughout body water, i.e. its apparent volume of distribution is about 50 litres in a 70 kg person
C Its use must be controlled by regular measurement of plasma concentration
D Concomitant use of a diuretic can reduce renal clearance of the drug, causing toxicity
E Nephrogenic diabetes insipidus may result from its use

19.19 Amphetamine

A acts by increasing the amount of noradrenaline stored in nerve endings throughout the nervous system
B has low potential for abuse
C in acute overdose can cause an acute psychotic state
D in chronic overdose can cause vasculitis
E is useful in narcolepsy

19.20 The following statements about caffeine and caffeine-containing drinks are correct:

A Tea, coffee and chocolate all contain caffeine
B Caffeine can stimulate mental activity above normal
C Caffeine causes a decrease in reaction time
D A cup of instant coffee contains about 80 mg of caffeine
E Clinically significant overdose of caffeine can occur with amounts in excess of 5 cups of coffee or 10 cups of tea a day

19.21 The following statements about xanthines are correct:

A   Aminophylline is effective for neonatal apnoea

B   Caffeine is useful primarily to relieve and prevent fatigue

C   Caffeine metabolism is dose-dependent

D   Caffeine in overdose may mimic an anxiety state

E   Drinking 5 cups of boiled coffee per day increases serum cholesterol by up to 10%

20 Epilepsy, parkinsonism and allied conditions

20.1   In the management of epilepsy

A   two drugs should be given together as initial therapy
B   patients must be persuaded of the importance of continuous medication
C   treatment must be life-long
D   it may be possible to discover and eliminate precipitating factors
E   the timing of medication should be adjusted if seizures occur only at a particular time of day or night

20.2   In the management of epilepsy

A   sudden cessation of treatment may result in status epilepticus
B   monitoring plasma concentration of drugs is useful in pregnancy
C   the majority of patients can be controlled on a single drug
D   two equal daily doses, morning and evening, are generally recommended
E   most patients can be relieved of their fits within one year of starting treatment

20.3   In epileptic women under treatment

A   there is a × 2.5 increase in the rate of malformations in their children

B   the physiological changes of pregnancy do not alter the pharmacokinetics of antiepilepsy drugs

C   drug therapy should be stopped during pregnancy

D   any malformation in their children is more likely to be due to the disease rather than the drugs

E   with drugs that accelerate the metabolism of oral contraceptives, a high dose oestrogen preparation should be used

20.4   In the treatment of epilepsy

A   carbamazepine or sodium valproate are first-choice drugs for major seizures

B   ethosuximide is a first-choice drug for absence attacks

C   paraldehyde is the first-choice drug for status epilepticus

D   when the dose is changed some drugs may take a week or more to reach a steady concentration in the plasma

E   adjustments of dosage require that a diary of seizures be kept

20.5   Phenytoin

A   plasma $t\frac{1}{2}$ is the same at all plasma concentrations

B   is subject only to first-order kinetics

C   enhances its own metabolism

D   is unlikely to cause drug interactions in a patient taking other medication

E   has a remarkably small range of adverse effects

20.6 **The following statements about antiepileptic drugs are correct:**

A Sodium valproate is a potent hepatic enzyme inducer
B In a patient taking sodium valproate blood coagulation should be examined before surgery is undertaken
C Vigabatrin acts by causing gamma-amino butyric acid (GABA) to accumulate in the brain
D Diazepam is effective in status epilepticus
E Lamotrigine is a useful adjuvant for generalised tonic-clonic seizures

20.7 **In Parkinson's disease**

A the basal ganglia are deficient in dopamine
B anticholinesterases improve movement
C reserpine replenishes dopamine stores
D chlorpromazine aggravates the condition
E amantadine improves movements by its dopaminergic and antimuscarinic effects

20.8 **Levodopa**

A is a metabolic product of dopamine
B penetrates poorly into the central nervous system
C is not metabolised in peripheral tissues
D may cause nausea
E may cause involuntary movements

20.9 **The following statements about levodopa and dopamine are correct:**

A Dopa decarboxylase inhibitors must enter the brain to be effective
B Dangerous hypertension may occur if levodopa is taken with a nonselective monoamine oxidase inhibitor
C Carbidopa is a dopamine agonist
D Tricylic antidepressants antagonise the effect of levodopa
E Metabolites of dopamine can interfere with some tests for phaeochromocytoma

20.10 Bromocriptine

A is a dopamine D_2-receptor antagonist
B has a longer plasma $t\frac{1}{2}$ than levodopa
C can cause psychiatric disturbances
D can cause postural hypotension
E may be used for patients who develop end-of-dose deterioration with levodopa

20.11 The following statements about apomorphine and selegiline are correct:

A Apomorphine is an agonist at dopamine D_1- and D_2-receptors
B Apomorphine may be used to treat the on-off phenomenon in Parkinson's disease
C Selegiline is a monoamine oxidase type A inhibitor
D Selegiline does not cause the hypertensive 'cheese' reaction
E Selegiline may be used to counteract end of dose akinesia

20.12 In the treatment of parkinsonism

A antimuscarinic drugs are particularly effective in relieving hypokinesia
B levodopa is particularly effective in reducing tremor
C amantadine is as effective as levodopa
D ankle oedema may be caused by amantadine
E due to neuroleptics, antimuscarinics are effective

20.13 In the treatment of Parkinson's disease

A levodopa initially restores 75% of patients to near normal function
B 25% of patients will still derive substantial or moderate benefit after 6 years of levodopa
C failure of initial response to levodopa questions the diagnosis
D rapid increment in dose is to be encouraged
E the 'on–off' phenomenon is worsened by increasing the frequency of dosing

20.14 The following statements are correct:

A Chorea may be alleviated by drugs that reduce the effect of dopamine

B Benign essential tremor is alleviated by alcohol

C Baclofen reduces muscle spasticity of central origin by its action as a GABA agonist

D Acute dystonic reactions due to neuroleptics should be treated with i.v. levodopa

E Botulinum toxin, injected locally, is effective for blepharospasm

20.15 In clinical tetanus

A treatment for convulsions may be initiated with chlorpromazine

B overtreatment with chlorpromazine may make convulsions worse

C α- and β-adrenoceptor blocking drugs benefit cardiovascular effects of tetanus toxin

D opioids are beneficial

E treatment with tubocurarine and artificial respiration should be used where there is laryngospasm

21 Anaesthesia and neuromuscular block

21.1 **The following statements about stages of anaesthesia are correct:**

A   Stage 1 sense of touch is retained and sense of hearing increased

B   In Stage 2 delirium may occur

C   In surgical anaesthesia (Stage 3) the corneal reflex is retained

D   Some degree of medullary paralysis occurs at all planes of Stage 3

E   Stages 1 and 2 are hardly recognisable with modern techniques

21.2 **The responsibility of the anaesthetist**

A   begins immediately before surgery when the patient arrives at the operating theatre

B   involves consideration of intercurrent illness

C   requires that he/she be informed of all drugs the patient may be receiving

D   commonly involves providing unconsciousness, analgesia and muscular relaxation with a separate drug for each purpose

E   ceases when patient leaves the operating theatre

21.3   Anaesthetic premedication involves considerations relating to

A   alertness
B   amnesia
C   analgesia
D   bronchial and salivary secretion
E   gastric contents

21.4   An anaesthetic for abdominal surgery may include

A   gradual induction by an inhaled agent
B   maintenance by an agent given intravenously
C   a halogenated agent
D   analgesia with an opioid given i.v.
E   muscular relaxation with tubocurarine

21.5   The following statements about anaesthetic techniques are correct:

A   Dissociative anaesthesia is a state of analgesia with light hypnosis
B   Dissociative anaesthesia is unsuitable at scenes of major accident
C   Neuroleptanalgesia is a state in which analgesia is effective and the patient remains cooperative
D   Neuroleptanalgesia can be provided by a combination of droperidol and fentanyl
E   A benzodiazepine can reliably be expected to provide retrograde amnesia for procedures such as endoscopy

21.6 **The following statements about the kinetics of inhalation anaesthetics are correct:**

A An agent that is highly soluble in blood, given at constant rate, provides a slow induction

B Nitrous oxide provides slow induction

C Diffusion hypoxia occurs when there is a flow of the anaesthetic agent from the alveoli to the blood

D Diffusion hypoxia occurs particularly with nitrous oxide when the agent is withdrawn

E Recovery from anaesthesia is fast if the agent is relatively insoluble in blood

21.7 **The following statements about halogenated anaesthetic agents are correct:**

A Halothane has a high blood/gas partition coefficient

B Halothane induces hepatic enzymes

C Enflurane is likely to cause diffusional hypoxia

D Prolonged use of enflurane may result in impaired renal function

E Isoflurane has the most favourable risk–benefit profile of the group

21.8 **Halothane**

A provides quick induction and recovery

B may cause cardiac dysrhythmias

C may cause jaundice if given repeatedly in the course of a few weeks

D should not be used if previous use has been followed by unexplained fever

E potentiates the effect of antihypertensive agents

21.9   Intravenous anaesthetics

  A provide slow induction
  B provide particularly quick recovery even after prolonged use
  C depend for their duration of effect on redistribution of drug in the body
  D depending on metabolism for their elimination can be expected to have a short duration of action
  E may be used to induce anaesthesia prior to administration of inhalational agents

21.10   Thiopentone

  A induces hypnosis and anaesthesia with analgesia
  B given i.v. causes brief apnoea
  C may cause laryngospasm during induction
  D has a plasma $t\frac{1}{2}$ of 9 minutes during the phase of distribution to the brain
  E has a plasma $t\frac{1}{2}$ of 9 hours after equilibration with fatty tissues

21.11   A neuromuscular blocking drug

  A may act by competition
  B may act by depolarisation
  C can be expected to impair consciousness
  D has its action reversed by an anticholinesterase in the case of suxamethonium
  E also blocks autonomic ganglia in the case of tubocurarine

21.12   Neuromuscular blocking drugs

  A may induce bronchospasm
  B carry no risk of awareness during surgery
  C are sufficiently selective to allow spontaneous respiration to be maintained in many cases
  D acting by competition are preferred for long procedures
  E acting by depolarisation may be associated with unduly prolonged paralysis

21.13 Neuromuscular blocking agents are useful in

A myasthenia gravis
B status epilepticus
C hypertension
D tetanus
E electroconvulsive therapy (ECT)

21.14 Baclofen

A does not cause objectionable sedation
B improves voluntary motor power
C may make the patient worse even if spasticity in the legs is reduced
D controls flexor spasms
E inhibits reflex activity in the spinal cord

21.15 Local anaesthetics

A act by altering sodium permeability of nerve cell membranes
B prevent initiation and propagation of the nerve impulse
C may be absorbed sufficiently (with topical application) to cause systemic toxicity
D affect first the larger (motor) nerve fibres and last the small (sensory) fibres
E have a stimulant effect on the central nervous system

21.16 Local anaesthetic

A action may be prolonged by addition of a vasodilator
B nerve block to an extremity (e.g. toe) should always be conducted with added adrenaline
C mixed with adrenaline is generally safe in a patient taking a monoamine oxidase inhibitor
D mixed with adrenaline can be dangerous in a patient with cardiovascular disease
E mixed with felypressin is preferable in patients with cardiovascular disease

21.17 Local anaesthetics

A   are usually effective within 5 minutes of application
B   have a useful duration of action of 1–1.5 hours
C   are most stable in the form of acid salts
D   of ester type may exhibit prolonged action where there is genetic defect
E   have an enhanced action in inflamed tissues

21.18 Local anaesthetic

A   overdose can cause convulsions
B   overdose can cause cardiovascular collapse
C   may be given i.v. to provide regional anaesthesia
D   may cause hypertension in the case of cocaine
E   must never be infiltrated around major peripheral nerves or near the spinal cord

21.19 The following statements about local anaesthetics are correct:

A   Lignocaine is useful in cardiac dysrhythmias
B   Prilocaine is less toxic than lignocaine
C   Prilocaine and lignocaine are components of EMLA (eutetic mixture of local anaesthetics)
D   Bupivacaine is preferred for obstetric epidural anaesthesia
E   Bupivacaine has a shorter duration of action than lignocaine

21.20 Cocaine

A   is effective on mucous membranes
B   enhances natural catecholamine effects
C   is not absorbed across mucous membranes
D   is abused for its central nervous system stimulation
E   overdose should be treated by adrenoceptor blocking drugs

21.21 **The following statements about the use of drugs in childbirth are correct:**

A Pethidine depresses fetal respiration more than morphine

B Naloxone antagonises both morphine and pethidine, given to mother or child

C Delay of gastric emptying due to opioids can be reversed by metoclopramide

D Diazepam dose must be carefully restricted as it is capable of depressing the newborn baby for several days

E Neuromuscular blocking drugs should be avoided for general anaesthesia

21.22 **The following statements about the interaction of anaesthetics with other drugs are correct:**

A A patient taking a monoamine oxidase inhibitor may safely be prescribed pethidine

B A patient under treatment for hypertension is liable to hypotension during general anaesthesia

C Antiepileptic drugs should be discontinued for a few days before anaesthesia

D Diuretic-induced hypokalaemia potentiates neuromuscular blocking drugs

E Aminoglycoside antibiotics antagonise neuromuscular blocking drugs

21.23 **The following statements about anaesthesia in special patient groups are correct:**

A Thiopentone induction is undesirable in patients with fixed cardiac output, e.g. mitral stenosis

B Patients with myasthenia gravis are intolerant of competitive neuromuscular blockers

C Morphine by injection is the preferred mode of premedication in children

D Dantrolene is the drug of choice for malignant hyperthermia

E In general, elderly patients require larger doses of anaesthetic agents

21.24 Factors which may influence the normal response to anaesthesia, including adjuvant drugs, include

A dystrophia myotonica
B porphyria
C sickle-cell disease
D the age of the patient
E raised intracranial pressure

22 Cholinergic and antimuscarinic (anticholinergic) drugs

22.1 **The following statements about cholinergic agents are correct:**

A The actions of acetylcholine at autonomic ganglia and the neuromuscular junction are described as nicotinic

B Pilocarpine inhibits cholinesterase

C Physostigmine blocks the actions of acetylcholine at nicotinic receptors

D Cholinergic drugs cause bronchodilation

E Pilocarpine lowers intraocular pressure in chronic simple glaucoma

22.2 **The following statements about cholinergic agents are correct:**

A Pilocarpine has a clinically useful miotic action

B Pilocarpine may be used to relieve dry mouth in patients taking large doses of an antimuscarinic drug

C The commonest adverse effect of pilocarpine is sweating

D Cholinergic drugs cause muscle fasciculation

E Amanita muscaria was highly valued by inhabitants of Eastern Siberia for its cerebral stimulant effects

22.3 **Cholinergic stimulation causes**

A intraocular pressure to rise

B sweating

C tachycardia

D reduced gut motility

E contraction of the bladder

22.4 **The following statements about anticholinesterases are correct:**

A Pseudocholinesterases metabolise substances other than acetylcholine

B Physostigmine lowers intraocular pressure

C Neostigmine may be used with atropine to reverse competitive neuromuscular block

D Pyridostigmine has fewer visceral effects than neostigmine

E Edrophonium has a long duration of action

22.5 **In anticholinesterase poisoning**

A due to organophosphorus insecticides, inhibition of cholinesterase is irreversible and recovery depends on formation of fresh enzyme

B bronchoconstriction may occur

C atropine should not be used

D due to organophosphorus insecticides, treatment with pralidoxime should be delayed for 24 hours

E recovery of plasma cholinesterase may take several weeks

22.6 **In myasthenia gravis**

A edrophonium given for diagnostic purposes should be accompanied by atropine to suppress unwanted visceral (muscarinic) effects

B with the Eaton–Lambert syndrome response to anticholinesterases is good

C a resistant myasthenic crisis may be improved by plasmapheresis to remove circulating antibodies

D edrophonium exaggerates a myasthenic crisis

E neuromuscular block is improved by atropine

22.7   In myasthenia gravis

A   neostigmine is preferred to pyridostigmine for the first dose of the day
B   thymectomy benefits most patients
C   azathioprine should not be used as a steroid sparing agent
D   prednisolone induces improvement or remission in 80% of cases
E   prednisolone is contraindicated when the disease is predominantly ocular

22.8   Atropine

A   antagonises all the effects of cholinergic drugs except those at autonomic ganglia and the neuromuscular junction
B   promotes sweating
C   relaxes smooth muscle
D   is used to treat glaucoma
E   inhibits milk production

22.9   Atropine

A   administered to the eye may interfere with normal pupillary responses for up to 2 weeks
B   reduces the heart rate
C   loosens viscid bronchial secretions
D   may induce urinary retention
E   should be avoided in cholinergic poisoning

22.10   Features of atropine poisoning include

A   mydriasis
B   hallucinations
C   hypothermia
D   coma
E   dry mouth

22.11 Anticholinergic drugs may be used to treat

A asthma
B colic
C urinary urgency incontinence
D vomiting
E heart block

22.12 Nicotine may be used therapeutically

A to abort premature labour
B to achieve controlled hypotension during surgery
C as an adjunct to counselling during tobacco withdrawal
D as either a gum or skin patches
E to suppress unwanted effects of anticholinesterases

23 Adrenergic mechanisms: (sympathomimetics, shock, hypotension)

23.1 **The following statements about the effects of adrenaline and noradrenaline are correct:**

A The classification of adrenoceptors is based on the observation that block of the whole range of actions of adrenaline could not be attained by a single drug

B There are two major classes of adrenoceptor

C α-adrenoceptor blocking drugs block the cardiac and vasodilator effects of adrenaline

D β-adrenoceptor blocking drugs block the vasoconstrictor effect of adrenaline and noradrenaline

E Relaxation of the smooth muscle of the bronchi and uterus is mediated by β-adrenoceptors

23.2 **Drugs may mimic or impair adrenergic mechanisms by**

A binding directly onto adrenoceptors

B discharging noradrenaline stored in nerve endings

C preventing reuptake into nerve endings of noradrenaline that has been released

D preventing destruction of noradrenaline in the nerve ending

E depleting noradrenaline stores in nerve endings

23.3 **Drugs may mimic or impair adrenergic mechanisms by**

A causing the nerve ending to synthesise a false transmitter

B acting in the central nervous system

C acting at parasympathetic nerve terminals

D acting as first messengers at adrenoceptors

E acting as second messengers at adrenoceptors

23.4 Physiological events mediated by α-adrenoceptors include

A increased heart rate
B hypokalaemia
C peripheral arteriolar constriction
D bronchoconstriction
E cardiac dysrhythmia

23.5 Physiological events mediated by β-adrenoceptors include

A mydriasis
B peripheral arteriolar dilation
C relaxation of pregnant myometrium
D voluntary muscle tremor
E increased myocardial contractility

23.6 The following statements about the action of sympathomimetics are correct:

A Adrenaline has almost exclusively β-adrenoceptor agonist actions
B Noradrenaline has an approximately equal mix of α-and β-adrenoceptor agonist actions
C Isoprenaline has predominantly α-adrenoceptor agonist actions
D Amphetamine acts indirectly by causing release of noradrenaline stored in nerve endings
E Dopamine acts not only on specific dopamine receptors but also on β-adrenoceptors

23.7 Catecholamines comprise

A adrenaline
B noradrenaline
C dopamine
D dobutamine
E salbutamol

23.8 Catecholamines

A are destroyed by monoamine oxidase
B released at nerve endings are at once destroyed by catechol-O-methyltransferase in the synaptic cleft
C are normally administered by mouth
D have a $t\frac{1}{2}$ of about two minutes
E may be administered i.m. or i.v.

23.9 The following statements about the action of sympathomimetics (i.v.) are correct:

A Noradrenaline infusion causes a rise of systolic and diastolic blood pressure with bradycardia
B Adrenaline infusion causes a rise of systolic and fall of diastolic blood pressure with tachycardia
C Isoprenaline causes little change in systolic and fall in diastolic blood pressure with tachycardia
D Dopamine causes cardiac stimulation with overall slight reduction in total peripheral resistance and increased renal blood flow
E Dobutamine has greater inotropic than chronotropic effects on the heart

23.10 Shock

A is a state of peripheral vascular hypoperfusion causing anoxic injury to vital organs
B may be caused by infections
C may be caused by loss of fluid from the circulation
D may be caused by cardiac injury
E is treated primarily by increasing peripheral vascular resistance with vasoconstrictor drugs

23.11 **When the needs of a patient in shock have been carefully defined, the following statements are correct:**

A Reduction of peripheral vascular resistance by α-adrenoceptor blocking drug may be useful

B Gelatin may be used to restore lost intravascular volume

C Dopamine or dobutamine provides a beneficial mix of adrenergic actions on heart and circulation

D Atropine relieves harmful bradycardia

E A vasodilator drug is indicated for a patient with low blood volume

24 Arterial hypertension, angina pectoris, myocardial infarction

24.1 Antihypertensive drugs may produce their effects by actions on

A   arteriole resistance vessels
B   venule capacitance vessels
C   adrenal cortex
D   central nervous system
E   blood volume

24.2 Antihypertensive drugs may block

A   ATP dependent K^+ channels
B α-adrenoceptors
C β-adrenoceptors
D   noradrenaline synthesis
E   noradrenaline release

24.3 Angiotensin converting enzyme (ACE) inhibitors

A   block the alteration of inactive angiotensin I to active angiotensin II
B   oppose the vasoconstrictor effect of angiotensin II
C   stimulate renal aldosterone production
D   should be avoided in patients taking aspirin
E   are more effective in lowering blood pressure in patients over 60 years than in younger patients

24.4 **The following statements about arterial antihypertensive and vasodilator drugs are correct:**

A Antihypertensives which cause vasodilatation need to be combined with a diuretic to prevent fluid retention

B Nitrates should not be used in patients with acute left ventricular failure due to hypertension

C Nifedipine causes less sympathetic activation than hydralazine when administered acutely as a capsule

D Vasodilators are the treatment of choice for the treatment of hypertension associated with a dissecting aortic aneurysm

E Diazoxide suppresses insulin secretion

24.5 **Glyceryl trinitrate**

A relieves an attack of angina pectoris by dilating the venous and arteriolar systems

B may be substituted by isosorbide dinitrate for prophylaxis of angina pectoris

C action lasts about 4 hours

D should be given at once if myocardial infarction is suspected

E is more effective for immediate pain relief than isosorbide dinitrate because it does not need to be metabolised

24.6 **When glyceryl trinitrate tablets are prescribed for angina pectoris the patient should be told**

A to take it to prevent pain

B to take it at onset of pain

C that if throbbing headache and palpitations occur the patient should seek immediate medical help

D that if pain is present 15 minutes later, it is not cardiac pain

E to keep the tablets in a warm humid place e.g. a shelf over the bath

24.7 Glyceryl trinitrate may usefully be prescribed as

A   a sublingual tablet
B   a tablet to swallow
C   an oral mucosal spray
D   an ointment
E   an intravenous infusion

24.8 The following vasodilator drugs are useful for relief or prevention of pain in stable angina:

A   Angiotensis converting enzyme inhibitors
B   Calcium channel blockers
C   Doxazosin
D   Hydralazine
E   Timolol

24.9 Diazoxide

A   is a thiazide
B   is a diuretic
C   is a vasodilator
D   is extensively bound to plasma protein
E   should be given intravenously very slowly

24.10 Amlodipine

A   is useful for long-term control of hypertension
B   causes sodium retention
C   is particularly useful for hypertension during childbirth (labour)
D   should not be given to patients with impaired left ventricular function
E   acts on arterioles (cardiac afterload) rather than on veins (cardiac preload)

24.11 Hydralazine

A may cause systemic lupus erythematosus
B should not be given with a diuretic
C is particularly suitable for sole treatment of hypertension
D characteristically causes bradycardia
E is a suitable drug for dissecting aortic aneurysm

24.12 In obstructive peripheral vascular disease

A drug therapy is more likely to be beneficial in arteriosclerosis than in vascular spasm
B if the skin of the leg becomes warmer it can be assumed flow to the muscles is similarly improved
C nocturnal muscle cramps occur and may be relieved by quinine
D a β-adrenoceptor blocker benefits
E any benefit from naftidofuryl may be due to metabolic changes in the muscle rather than to vasodilatation

24.13 The following statements about α-adrenoceptor blocking drugs are correct:

A Phentolamine is contraindicated for adrenergic hypertensive crises
B Phenoxybenzamine is an irreversible antagonist
C Those that block α_1- and α_2-adrenoceptors may be associated with troublesome tachycardia
D Prazosin may cause hypotension after the initial dose
E Labetalol has both α- and β-adrenoceptor blocking actions

24.14 Most β-adrenoceptor blocking drugs cause

A reduction of heart rate
B increased myocardial contractility
C reduced peripheral blood flow
D bronchoconstriction
E reduced blood flow to the liver and kidneys

24.15 β-adrenoceptor blocking drugs

A increase myocardial oxygen consumption
B with some agonist effect are particularly useful in patients with impaired left ventricular function
C with membrane stabilising effect are more useful as antidysrhythmics than as antihypertensives
D are useful when blood pressure must be lowered within a few hours
E selective for cardiac β_1-receptors can safely be used in asthmatics

24.16 β-adrenoceptor blocking drugs that are lipid soluble

A readily enter the central nervous system
B readily allow the duration of β-adrenoceptor blockade to be predicted from the $t^{\frac{1}{2}}$
C may show less predictable plasma concentrations than do those that are water soluble
D are preferred if there is renal insufficiency
E may cause sleep disturbance

24.17 β-adrenoceptor blocking drugs are used in

A essential hypertension
B anxiety
C hypothyroidism
D cardiac dysrhythmias
E glaucoma

24.18 Patients taking a β-adrenoceptor blocking drug may experience

A exacerbation of existing heart block
B precipitation of heart failure
C incapacity for vigorous exercise
D cold extremities
E hypoglycaemia if they are diabetic

24.19 **The following statements about angiotensin converting enzyme (ACE) inhibitors and losartan, an angiotensin receptor antagonist, are correct:**

A   ACE inhibitor therapy for a patient taking a diuretic is best initiated with a morning dose

B   Losartan diminishes angiotensin reuptake into sympathetic nerves

C   ACE inhibitors reduce blood pressure by lowering cardiac output

D   Losartan is useful as a replacement for an ACE inhibitor when this causes cough

E   ACE inhibitors postpone the onset of diabetic nephropathy

24.20 **Clonidine**

A   acts on β-adrenoceptors in the brain

B   acts on presynaptic α_2-adrenoceptors at the sympathetic nerve ending

C   reduces noradrenaline secretion

D   withdrawal, if sudden, may be followed by dangerous hypertension

E   causes sedation and dry mouth

24.21 **Methyldopa**

A   acts through the formation of a false sympathetic transmitter

B   acts primarily on peripheral nerves

C   is effective for hypertension in pregnancy

D   may cause haemolytic anaemia

E   may cause depression

24.22 **Angina pectoris pain not adequately controlled by (short-term) glyceryl trinitrate may respond to**

A   calcium channel block

B   β-adrenoceptor block

C   α-adrenoceptor block

D K^+ channel activation (nicorandil)

E   a statin hypolipidaemic

24.23 **The following statements about treatment of arterial hypertension are correct:**

A The value of antihypertensive drugs resides chiefly in their ability to prevent stroke and cardiac failure

B First dose hypotension is unusual with drugs that do not alter venous tone

C Elderly people benefit less than young from reduction of blood pressure

D Elderly hypertensives respond better to angiotensin converting enzyme inhibitors than do the young

E Aspirin should be given to all hypertensive patients to reduce the risk of myocardial infarction

24.24 **In the control of hypertension**

A an angiotensin converting enzyme inhibitor is usefully combined with a diuretic

B a β-adrenoceptor blocker is safely and effectively combined with a calcium channel blocker

C ankle oedema caused by a calcium channel blocker should be treated by a diuretic

D use of potassium supplements is preferred to that of a potassium-retaining diuretic to conserve body potassium

E methyldopa is a drug of choice for initial therapy

24.25 **Long term thiazide diuretic use can cause**

A hyperkalaemia

B impaired male sexual function

C impaired glucose tolerance

D gout

E Raynaud's phenomenon

24.26 Emergency control of severe hypertension by parenteral therapy is indicated in

A   dissecting aortic aneurysm
B   hypertensive encephalopathy
C   acute left ventricular failure due to hypertension
D   accelerated phase hypertension
E   eclampsia

24.27 In hypertension of pregnancy

A   a diuretic is preferred
B   hydralazine is acceptable in the first trimester
C   atenolol in the first trimester may cause small babies
D   labetalol is a useful and safe treatment
E   magnesium infusion is used to treat eclamptic fits

24.28 The following statements about phaeochromocytoma are correct:

A   Most antihypertensive drugs interfere with the biochemical tests for this condition
B   In a hypertensive emergency β-adrenoceptor blocking drug must be given first
C   In a hypertensive emergency phentolamine is a drug of choice
D   Phenoxybenzamine treatment should be given for several weeks before surgery to permit vascular expansion
E   Blood pressure response to an α-adrenoceptor blocking drug is the most sensitive confirmation of the diagnosis

25 Cardiac dysrhythmia and failure

25.1 The following statements about cardiac cells are correct:

A The atrioventricular node discharges automatically 45 times per minute

B The sinoatrial node discharges automatically 25 times per minute

C Altered rate of automatic discharge may be a cause of cardiac dysrhythmia

D In its phases of polarisation, the cardiac cell is hyperexcitable during phases 1 and 2

E Cardiac dysrhythmia may result from impaired conduction leading to the formation of re-entry circuits

25.2 The following statements about the classification of antidysrhythmic drugs are correct:

A Class 1 drugs possess membrane stabilising activity

B Class 1A drugs shorten refractoriness

C Class 1B drugs lengthen refractoriness

D Class II drugs block slow calcium channels

E Class III drugs reduce the activity of the sympathetic nervous system

25.3 Quinidine

A depresses myocardial contractility

B reduces vagal nerve activity on the heart

C is used for resistant supraventricular tachycardia

D lowers plasma digoxin concentration

E should be used alone to treat atrial flutter

25.4 Disopyramide

A possesses membrane stabilising activity
B prolongs the cardiac refractory period
C is contraindicated for patients with Wolff-Parkinson-White syndrome
D has a positive inotropic effect
E should be avoided in patients with glaucoma

25.5 Lignocaine

A possesses membrane stabilising activity
B reduces the cardiac refractory period
C is not given orally because it is not absorbed from the gastrointestinal tract
D is particularly effective for supraventricular dysrhythmias
E may cause convulsions

25.6 The following statements about cardiac antidysrhythmic drugs are correct:

A Mexiletine should be used for supraventricular tachycardias
B Adenosine may help to distinguish the cause of 'broad QRS complex' tachycardias
C Adenosine is used to treat supraventricular (re-entrant) tachycardias
D Flecainide is used mainly for ventricular dysrhythmias
E Sotalol has class III but no class I antidysrhythmic activity

25.7 The following statements about cardiac antidysrhythmic drugs are correct:

A Esmolol is used for parenteral treatment of dysrhythmias because of its long duration of action
B Propranolol in overdose may cause heart block
C Emergency treatment of dysrhythmias with amiodarone requires i.v. infusion because its $t_{\frac{1}{2}}$ is short
D Thyroid function should be checked before a patient begins treatment with amiodarone
E The dose of warfarin should be decreased in patients who receive amiodarone

25.8 **The following statements about calcium channel blocking drugs are correct:**

A Verapamil has a positive inotropic effect
B Diltiazem is safe to use where there is sick sinus syndrome
C Verapamil used with β-adrenoceptor blocker may cause cardiac failure in patients with depressed myocardial contractility
D Amlodipine is safe to use in patients with cardiac failure
E Nifedipine is effective for supraventricular dysrhythmias

25.9 **Stimulation of the vagus nerve**

A causes tachycardia due to its effect on the sinoatrial node
B accelerates conduction in the atrioventricular tissue
C is counteracted by atropine
D shortens the refractory period of atrial muscle
E decreases myocardial excitability

25.10 **Reflex stimulation of the vagus nerve for cardiac dysrhythmia may be produced by**

A inviting patients to put their fingers down their throats
B pressing on both carotid sinuses simultaneously
C the Valsalva manoeuvre
D the Muller procedure
E swallowing ice-cream

25.11 **Stimulation of the sympathetic nervous system**

A causes tachycardia due to increased rate of discharge of the sinoatrial node
B increases conductivity in the His-Purkinje system
C decreases force of cardiac contraction
D shortens the cardiac refractory period
E may be reproduced in the heart by administration of isoprenaline

25.12 Digoxin

A increases the excitability of the myocardium
B increases the contractility of the myocardium
C has its action terminated mainly by metabolism in the liver
D has a plasma $t\frac{1}{2}$ of less than 5 hours
E provides benefit in atrial fibrillation by increasing the force of cardiac contraction

25.13 Digoxin toxicity

A is strongly suggested by an ectopic dysrhythmia accompanied by heart block
B is more likely in the elderly
C may take the form of abnormal colour vision
D may explain gynaecomastia
E may explain mental confusion

25.14 Digoxin

A should be given in a lower dose if verapamil is also administered
B overdose responds well to treatment by dialysis
C overdose causing dysrhythmia responds to phenytoin
D overdose may be treated by infusion of specific digoxin-binding antibody fragments
E in severe overdose causes hyperkalaemia

25.15 The principal site of antidysrhythmic action of

A β-adrenoceptor blockers is the ventricle
B digoxin is the sinoatrial and atrioventricular nodes
C verapamil is the bundle of His
D atropine is the ventricle
E mexiletine is the atrium

25.16 Paroxysmal supraventricular tachycardia

A may be terminated by vagal stimulation
B if accompanied by atrioventricular block should be treated with verapamil
C may be treated with digoxin
D may be treated with adenosine
E may be prevented with a β-adrenoceptor blocker

25.17 In atrial fibrillation

A when conversion to sinus rhythm is urgent, direct current (DC) shock is preferred
B conversion to sinus rhythm should be attempted particularly if the left atrium is enlarged
C treatment with quinidine alone may give rise to a dangerous increase in ventricular rate
D amiodarone may be used for conversion to sinus rhythm
E rapid ventricular rate should be controlled by digoxin

25.18 The following statements about cardiac dysrhythmia are correct:

A Atrial ectopic beats may respond to reduced intake of xanthine-containing drinks
B With atrial tachycardia accompanied by A-V block, the cause may be digoxin
C Digoxin is the drug of choice for supraventricular tachycardia associated with the Wolff-Parkinson-White syndrome
D Lignocaine is effective in suppressing ventricular premature beats after myocardial infarction
E Amiodarone is effective treatment for recurrent ventricular tachycardia

25.19 In cardiac failure

A dilation of the heart helps temporarily to sustain cardiac output
B the heart and brain receive blood diverted from skeletal muscle
C most patients die from dysrhythmia
D diuretics lower excessive venous filling pressure
E nitrates stimulate myocardial contraction

25.20 In cardiac failure

A diuretic therapy does not benefit the symptom of fatigue
B the Starling curve predicts that, when the condition is advanced, cardiac output falls as filling pressure rises
C nitrates act partly by reducing preload
D angiotensin converting enzyme (ACE) inhibitors act by reducing preload and afterload
E ACE inhibitor therapy is best initiated with captopril

25.21 In cardiac failure

A ACE inhibitors improve symptoms but not survival
B digoxin is of no benefit in the long term for patients in sinus rhythm
C ACE inhibitors reduce the neurohumoral response to excessive diuresis
D with low output, the inotropic action of dobutamine may be useful in short term management
E dopamine may usefully increase renal blood flow in the short term

25.22 In heart failure, vasodilators

A can usefully be added to a diuretic
B relieve cardiac preload
C relieve cardiac afterload
D may reduce survival
E in use include enalapril and isosorbide dinitrate

26 Hyperlipidaemias

26.1 **The following statements about lipoproteins are correct:**

A High density lipoproteins (HDL) are protective against ischaemic heart disease

B Low density lipoproteins (LDL) constitute the major system for delivery of cholesterol to the tissues in man

C Endogenous triglyceride is carried in the circulation bound to very low density lipoproteins (VLDL)

D The lowest plasma cholesterol concentration that is associated with cardiovascular risk is 5.2 mmol/l

E Any fall in intracellular cholesterol leads to an increased expression of LDL receptors

26.2 **In the treatment of hyperlipidaemia**

A diet alone cannot be expected to produce improvement

B statins reduce circulating low density lipoproteins (LDL) by causing an up-regulation of hepatic LDL receptors

C fibrates reduce plasma triglyceride concentrations to a relatively greater degree than cholesterol

D cholestyramine may aggravate hypertriglyceridaemia

E patients with familial hypercholesterolaemia usually need an ion-exchange resin in addition to dietary advice

26.3 **The following statements about lipid-lowering therapy are correct:**

A Simvastatin causes a 30% reduction in total mortality in patients who have previously had a myocardial infarction

B Simvastatin reduces death from coronary artery disease by about 40% in patients who have previously had a myocardial infarction

C Treatment with pravastatin of 1000 men with LDL cholesterol 4–6 mmol/l is estimated to prevent myocardial infarction in 20 subjects per year

D Nicotinic acid may cause pallor of the skin

E α-tocopherol (vitamin E) may reduce the harmful effects of saturated fats in the arteries by preventing the oxidation of LDL

27 Kidney and urinary tract

27.1 **The following statements about renal physiology are correct:**

A Each day the body produces a maximum of 20 l of glomerular filtrate

B 65% of filtered sodium is reabsorbed isotonically by the proximal tubule

C Chloride is actively transported from the tubular fluid to the interstitial fluid in the thick segment of the ascending limb of the loop of Henle

D Interstitial fluid tonicity is high in the cortex and low in the medulla

E The ascending limb of the loop of Henle is impermeable to water

27.2 **Diuresis may result from**

A increase in cardiac output

B intravenous infusion of a low molecular weight non-electrolyte hypertonic solution

C inhibition of antidiuretic hormone secretion

D drug action on renal glomeruli

E stimulation of renal tubular carbonic anhydrase

27.3   In the kidney diuretic drugs act at the

A   proximal tubule by inhibiting active reabsorption of chloride

B   ascending limb of the loop of Henle by inhibiting active transport of water

C   cortical diluting segment by preventing sodium reabsorption

D   distal tubule by inhibiting the action of antidiuretic hormone

E   collecting tubule by inhibiting the action of aldosterone

27.4   The principal renal site of action of

A   triamterene is in the ascending limb of the loop of Henle

B   spironolactone is in the descending limb of the loop of Henle

C   frusemide is in the proximal tubule

D   osmotic diuretics is in the distal tubule

E   thiazides is in the cortical diluting segment

27.5   The following statements about the action of diuretics in the kidney are correct:

A   Loop diuretics diminish the osmotic gradient between medulla and cortex

B   Diuretics that act in the loop of Henle have a lower maximal effect than do drugs that act on the cortical diluting segment

C   Diuretics that act in the cortical diluting segment increase the osmotic gradient between medulla and cortex

D   Diuretics that act in the distal tubule have a weak natriuretic effect

E   Thiazides usually remain effective even at glomerular filtration rates below 20 ml/min

27.6 Diuretic drugs may be used to treat

A angioedema
B hypercalcaemia
C idiopathic hypercalciuria
D the syndrome of inappropriate antidiuretic hormone secretion
E nephrogenic diabetes insipidus

27.7 The following statements about high efficacy diuretics are correct:

A Frusemide is effective when the glomerular filtration rate is less than 10 ml/min
B Part of the effect of frusemide in relieving acute pulmonary oedema is due to vasodilatation
C The diuretic action of a single dose of bumetanide lasts 24 hours
D Ethacrynic acid may cause deafness
E Pancreatitis is a recognised adverse effect of frusemide

27.8 Thiazide diuretics

A are preferred to the loop diuretics for the treatment of hypertension
B raise potassium excretion to an important extent
C are uricosuric
D may cause thrombocytopenia
E are effective antihypertensives partly due to reduction of peripheral vascular resistance

27.9 The following statements about potassium-sparing diuretics are correct:

A Spironolactone has low therapeutic efficacy when used alone
B Spironolactone may cause gynaecomastia
C Spironolactone may cause hyperkalaemia in patients whose renal function is impaired
D Spironolactone may usefully be combined with triamterene
E Amiloride antagonises the action of aldosterone

27.10   **The following statements about minimising potassium depletion are correct:**

A   A good dietary intake of potassium is effective
B   Potassium tablets may cause gastrointestinal irritation
C   The loop diuretics cause a smaller fall in serum potassium that the thiazides for equivalent diuretic effect
D   Amiloride accelerates potassium loss
E   Combining a potassium-sparing with a potassium-losing drug is effective

27.11   **Hyperkalaemia**

A   is a particular risk if a potassium-sparing diuretic is used in a patient with impaired renal function
B   if severe may require dialysis for correction
C   increases if sodium bicarbonate is given
D   can be corrected by infusion of glucose and insulin
E   causing ECG changes is an indication to give calcium gluconate

27.12   **Adverse effects of diuretics include**

A   magnesium deficiency
B   chronic hypovolaemia
C   hypoglycaemia
D   sexual impotence
E   gout

27.13   **The following statements about osmotic diuretics are correct:**

A   Osmotic diuretics are large molecular weight substances
B   Osmotic diuretics lower intracranial pressure primarily by inducing diuresis
C   Intravenous mannitol can lower intraocular pressure
D   Osmotic diuretics act mainly in the collecting tubule where they prevent the reabsorption of water
E   Urine volume increases according to the load of osmotic diuretic

27.14 Acetazolamide

A is a carbonic anhydrase inhibitor
B causes a metabolic acidosis
C has diuretic activity
D cures acute mountain sickness by shifting the dissociation curve of O_2 from haemoglobin
E may be used to treat epilepsy

27.15 Cation-exchange resins

A are as effective diuretics as are thiazides
B are effective for the correction of hyperkalaemia
C of sodium phase are preferred for patients with cardiac failure
D of calcium phase should be avoided in patients with multiple myeloma
E may be given rectally

27.16 When diuretic drugs are used

A changes in body weight are useful in monitoring the dose
B restriction of dietary salt enhances their value in removal of oedema
C overdiuresis is usually suggested by rising blood urea concentration
D short courses of frusemide with metolazone are useful for resistant oedema
E to treat hepatic ascites, vigorous depletion of sodium is mandatory

27.17 The following statements about alteration of urine pH are correct:

A Alkalinisation may be achieved by oral potassium citrate
B Alkalinisation encourages the growth of *Escherichia coli*
C Alkalinisation prevents urate stone formation
D Acidification increases urinary elimination of paracetamol
E Acidification increases urinary elimination of salicylate

27.18 **The kidney may be damaged by**

    A gold
    B amphotericin
    C calciferol
    D cyclosporin
    E aminoglycosides

27.19 **Substances that may precipitate in the urine and obstruct the urinary tract include**

    A urate
    B methotrexate
    C citrate
    D calcium
    E allopurinol

27.20 **When prescribing a drug that is renally eliminated for a patient with renal impairment**

    A alteration of the initial (priming or loading) dose is generally unnecessary
    B the creatinine clearance is a useful guide to dosage
    C the normal maintenance dose may be given if the drug is metabolised to inactive products
    D the normal maintenance dose may be given provided the interval between doses is increased
    E the time to reach a steady state plasma concentration will be the same as in patients with normal renal function

27.21 **Drugs that are eliminated almost exclusively by the kidney include**

    A atenolol
    B digoxin
    C penicillin
    D rifampicin
    E warfarin

27.22 **Drugs that may be used in normal dose for patients with renal impairment include**

A amiodarone
B gentamicin
C paracetamol
D amoxycillin
E metformin

27.23 **Drugs that require close monitoring when used for patients with renal impairment include**

A doxycycline
B diazepam
C propranolol
D lithium
E pethidine

27.24 **The following statements about micturition are correct:**

A Flavoxate benefits urinary frequency by relaxing bladder smooth muscle
B Antimuscarinic drugs alleviate incontinence due to detrusor instability
C Imipramine is effective for nocturnal urinary incontinence
D Androgens applied locally to the vagina may benefit urinary incontinence due to atrophy of the urethral epithelium in women
E Activation of α_1-adrenoceptors causes the smooth muscle of the internal urethral sphincter to contract

27.25 **In the treatment of the symptoms of benign prostatic hypertrophy**

A indoramin benefits by blocking β-adrenoceptors
B prazosin acts by blocking α_1-adrenoceptors
C finasteride is rapidly effective at relieving symptoms
D finasteride acts by inhibiting the conversion of testosterone to dihydrotestosterone in the prostate
E finasteride increases libido

28 Respiratory system

28.1   Cough

A   that is due to a cause above the larynx often responds to a demulcent

B   that is due to a cause below the larynx often responds to water aerosol and benzoin inhalation

C   is reduced by opioids

D   is improved by antihistamines through block of histamine H_1-receptors

E   when intractable, may be relieved by lignocaine administered by nebuliser

28.2   The following statements about mucus and mucolytics are correct:

A   Iodides reduce mucus viscosity

B   Acetylcysteine increases sputum viscosity

C   Dornase alfa should be used only for patients with cystic fibrosis

D   Sputum viscosity may be lowered by rehydrating a patient

E   Mucolytics can cause gastrointestinal symptoms

28.3 The following statements about respiratory stimulation are correct:

A Respiratory stimulation is usually necessary in the management of an acute asthmatic attack

B Respiratory stimulation, as a short term measure, may avoid the need for assisted ventilation in patients with acute ventilatory failure due to exacerbation of chronic lung disease

C Doxapram has a larger margin between therapeutic and toxic doses than do other respiratory stimulants

D Patients with epilepsy may safely be given respiratory stimulants

E Aminophylline can provide useful respiratory stimulation for apnoeic premature infants

28.4 Oxygen

A should be used in low concentration for young patients with status asthmaticus

B in arterial blood at a partial pressure of 6.7 kPa is adequate to maintain tissue oxygenation in *chronically* hypoxic patients

C should not be used in high concentration (60%) even for short periods for patients with pulmonary embolism lest the hypoxic drive for respiration be removed

D must normally be used in concentrations exceeding 28% to provide adequate therapy for patients with infective exacerbations of chronic obstructive lung disease

E as continuous long-term (domiciliary) therapy improves survival in patients with severe persistent hypoxia and cor pulmonale due to chronic bronchitis and emphysema

28.5 Histamine

A acts principally as a systemic hormone
B causes capillaries to dilate
C inhibits gastric secretion
D causes bronchial muscle to relax
E causes itch

28.6 Some or all of the consequences of histamine release in the body can be opposed or prevented by

A adrenaline
B cimetidine
C astemizole
D terbinafine
E sodium cromoglycate

28.7 The histamine H_1-receptor antagonists are used for their sedative and other actions

A as hypnotics
B to treat Parkinson's disease
C as antitussives
D to treat acute urticaria
E to treat peptic ulcer

28.8 The following statements about histamine H_1-receptor antagonists are correct:

A Histamine H_1-receptor antagonists generally are competitive inhibitors of the action of histamine
B At therapeutic doses astemizole exhibits insurmountable antagonism of the action of histamine
C Histamine H_1-receptor antagonists are more effective if used before histamine has been liberated
D Astemizole has a rapid onset of action
E Promethazine is free from sedative effects

28.9 The following statements about allergic states are correct:

A In hay fever, rebound swelling of the nasal mucous membrane occurs when topical vasoconstrictor medication is stopped

B In severe angioedema, s.c. adrenaline provides quickest relief

C In cold urticaria combined histamine H_1- and H_2-receptor antagonism may be needed to block fully the vascular effects

D Hereditary angioedema does not respond to antihistamines and should be treated with fresh frozen plasma

E Adrenal steroids provide benefit by suppressing the effects on cells of antigen-antibody reactions

28.10 In asthma

A the principal inflammatory bronchoconstrictor mediator is histamine

B early in an attack hyperventilation maintains the paO_2 and keeps the $paCO_2$ low

C immediate reactions to inhaled allergens occur in non-atopic persons

D adult onset asthma is often not attributable to any known allergen

E some patients develop wheeze that regularly follows within a few minutes of exercise

28.11 In asthma

A anxiety is best alleviated by propranolol

B leukotriene antagonists, e.g. zileuton, may reduce corticosteroid use

C β-adrenoceptor agonists are preferred therapy

D hyposensitisation to allergens should normally be undertaken

E drugs with antimuscarinic action may be beneficial

28.12 Sodium cromoglycate

A is effective in the management of an acute attack of asthma
B is of no use in asthmatic children
C is normally given by the oral route
D is useful as eye-drops for hay fever
E causes drowsiness

28.13 Theophylline

A $t\frac{1}{2}$ is increased in patients with severe cardiopulmonary disease
B potentiates the response to adrenoceptor agonists, e.g. salbutamol, by inhibiting the breakdown of cyclic AMP
C in overdose causes cardiac dysrhythmia
D by suppository at night is effective for 'morning dippers'
E should be given in reduced dose by the intravenous route for an acute asthmatic attack if the patient has received the drug in the previous 24 hours

28.14 The following statements about the treatment of asthma are correct:

A Failure to respond to a metered dose aerosol is often due to improper technique of its use
B Ipratropium by metered dose aerosol may benefit elderly intrinsic asthmatics and patients with chronic obstructive airways disease
C Reduced hypothalamic-pituitary-adrenal responsiveness is a significant problem with the use of inhaled corticosteroids
D Inhaled corticosteroid may cause oropharyngeal candidiasis
E Adrenal suppression with oral corticosteroid may be minimised by giving it as a single evening dose

28.15 In status asthmaticus

A   salbutamol may be given by nebulised aerosol
B   ipratropium may be given by nebulised aerosol
C   hydrocortisone i.v. is preferred to oral prednisolone for initial therapy for very sick patients
D   humidified oxygen should be given
E   morphine provides useful sedation

28.16 The following statements about the use of β-adrenoceptor agonists in asthma are correct:

A   Salbutamol may cause hypokalaemia
B   About 20% of an inhaled dose of salbutamol is absorbed systemically and can cause cardiovascular effects
C   Salmeterol has a longer duration of action than other β_2 agonists
D   Salmeterol is particularly useful in the prevention of nocturnal asthma
E   Salmeterol should be reserved for the treatment of acute attacks

28.17 In the British Thoracic Society Guidelines for the Treatment of Asthma

A   step 2 requires regular use of an anti-inflammatory agent
B   salmeterol is recommended as an alternative to a corticosteroid
C   sodium cromoglycate is an alternative to a corticosteroid in step 2
D   oral prednisolone may be needed in patients whose peak expiratory flow rate is <80% of predicted despite high-dose inhaled corticosteroid
E   theophyllines (methylxanthine) are not recommended

29 Drugs and haemostasis

29.1   Vitamin K

A   is necessary for the formation of factor IX in the liver
B   requires bile for its absorption
C   given i.m. may cause childhood cancer
D   is required for the formation of the anticoagulant proteins C and S
E   deficiency may occur as a result of small intestine resection

29.2   The following statements about vitamin K preparations are correct:

A   Menadiol sodium phosphate may cause haemolytic anaemia
B   Phytomenadione is the most rapidly effective preparation of vitamin K
C   It is best to use menadiol sodium phosphate for treating hypoprothrombinaemia in neonates
D   Hypoprothrombinaemia due to intestinal malabsorption should be treated with phytomenadione
E   There is a danger of circulatory collapse if phytomenadione is given intravenously

29.3 Warfarin

A competitively inhibits vitamin K epoxide reductase

B can be expected to achieve effective anticoagulant protection in 72 hours

C treatment, when initiated, may lead to a transient hypercoagulable state

D should be avoided in early pregnancy because it may cause skeletal disorder in the fetus

E is a racemic mixture in which the S form is 4 times more active than the R form

29.4 In anticoagulant treatment with warfarin

A skin necrosis may result

B an International Normalised Ratio (INR) of 3.0–4.5 is advised for patients with recurrent deep vein thrombosis

C the incidence of major haemorrhage is 4–8%

D treatment of bleeding by phytomenadione i.v. renders the patient refractory to warfarin for 2 weeks

E the drug should on no account be stopped abruptly because of the risk of rebound thromboembolism

29.5 In patients taking warfarin the following statements are correct:

A Cardiac dysrhythmias should be treated with amiodarone rather than disopyramide

B Convulsions should be treated with phenytoin rather than sodium valproate

C Infections should be treated with metronidazole rather than a cephalosporin

D Depression may be treated with tricyclic antidepressants

E Benzodiazepines may be used to treat anxiety

29.6 Heparin

A was discovered by a medical student in the course of physiological research on blood clotting

B occurs in mast cells

C greatly enhances the activity of naturally occurring antithrombin III

D is readily absorbed from the gastrointestinal tract

E effect is immediately antagonised by protamine sulphate

29.7 In treatment with heparin

A low molecular weight preparations provide effective prophylaxis for deep vein thrombosis in once daily administrations

B optimum therapy is provided if the kaolin-cephalin clotting time (KCCT) is in the range 2.5–3.5 times control

C administration of 5000 units s.c. 8 hourly does not require monitoring of the KCCT

D thrombocytopenia with arterial thromboemboli may occur

E osteoporosis may develop in patients on therapeutic doses for more than 6 months

29.8 Anticoagulant treatment in established venous thrombosis

A should be continued for as long as 6 months if there is evidence of pulmonary embolus

B is unnecessary in the case of small distal thrombi

C is always preferred to streptokinase for thrombus in a large proximal vein

D is contraindicated in the presence of severe uncontrolled hypertension

E is more effective than treatment with an antiplatelet drug (aspirin)

29.9 Anticoagulant therapy

A in the long term should be considered for a patient with chronic atrial fibrillation

B in the long term should be considered for a patient with an enlarged left atrium

C with heparin should not be used for a patient with unstable angina

D should be used for most cases of intermittent claudication

E after myocardial infarction reduces the risk of mural thromboemboli

29.10 In the process of fibrinolysis

A plasminogen is a precursor of fibrin

B streptokinase acts as an inhibitor of plasmin

C alteplase acts as a tissue type plasminogen activator

D tranexamic acid blocks plasminogen binding to fibrin

E plasmin formation normally takes place on the fibrin surface rather than within the circulating blood

29.11 Coronary artery thrombolysis

A should be initiated at least 12 h after the onset of chest pain

B with anistreplase may be given by mouth

C shows substantial differences between different agents in terms of survival

D is contraindicated in a patient with a recent stroke

E is contraindicated in a patient with severe uncontrolled hypertension

29.12 Coronary artery thrombolysis

A may lead to cardiac dysrhythmias

B may cause multiple microemboli

C can be expected to lead to bleeding severe enough to require transfusion in 5% of cases

D with streptokinase is unlikely to lead to anaphylactic reactions if re-use takes place within 5 days

E may be useful in persisting unstable angina

29.13 The following statements about blood platelet activity are correct:

A Intact vascular endothelium does not attract platelets because of the high concentration of prostacyclin in the intima

B Thromboxane is derived mainly from platelets

C Dipyridamole reduces platelet activity by increasing cyclic AMP concentration

D Low dose aspirin (75 mg) selectively reduces synthesis of thromboxane A_2, without significantly impairing prostacyclin formation

E Dextrans, e.g. dextran 70, prolong the bleeding time

29.14 Aspirin

A should be given indefinitely to patients who have survived myocardial infarction

B alone is adequate treatment for unstable angina

C with dipyridamole improves the patency rates of arterial grafts

D should be given indefinitely to patients with transient ischaemic attacks

E acts by irreversible inhibition of prostaglandin G/H synthase

29.15 The following statements about haemostatics and haemophilia are correct:

A Adrenaline is only useful in epistaxis if given by systemic injection

B Fibrin glue can be used to secure surgical haemostasis on a large raw surface

C Tranexamic acid is of no value in the treatment of a haemophilic patient who has bled after tooth extraction

D Ethamsylate given systemically reduces bleeding in menorrhagia

E Desmopressin (DDAVP) usefully increases factor VIII and IX activity in mild to moderate haemophilia

30 Cellular disorders and anaemias

30.1   Iron

A   is transported in the body bound to ferritin
B   in haemoglobin accounts for less than $\frac{1}{3}$ of total body iron
C   released from destroyed erythrocytes is mostly excreted in the urine
D   intake in the diet of an average Western human is 10–15 mg a day
E   loss with menses amounts to about 30 mg/period

30.2   Absorption of iron from the gut

A   is greater in an anaemic than in a normal human
B   is enhanced by ascorbic acid
C   is more efficient if it is in ferric form
D   is reduced by formation of phosphate salts
E   takes place mostly in the upper small intestine

30.3   In iron deficiency

A   the measurement of transferrin in the blood gives a good indication of the body's iron stores
B   replacement with oral iron should continue for 3 months after the blood haemoglobin concentration has reached normal
C   failure of response to oral iron is unlikely to be due to lack of compliance by the patient
D   25 mg of ferrous sulphate daily by mouth will produce a rise of 1% of haemoglobin per day
E   it is important to give an initial loading dose of whatever iron preparation is used

30.4 In iron therapy

A oral iron may safely be continued during a course of i.m. iron sorbitol

B liquid iron formulations may stain the teeth

C tests for occult blood in the faeces are not generally interfered with

D intramuscular iron sorbitol may cause the urine to turn black

E previously undetected folic acid deficiency is sometimes unmasked in the course of treatment

30.5 In acute iron poisoning

A symptoms are steadily progressive during the first 24 hours

B convulsions are to be expected within $\frac{1}{2}$ hour of ingestion

C cardiovascular collapse is a feature

D gastrointestinal obstruction is a late complication

E raw egg and milk will help to bind iron until medical help is available

30.6 Desferrioxamine

A is excreted in the urine giving it a reddish colour

B is of little or no value in acute iron poisoning

C given i.v. can cause adult respiratory distress syndrome

D is indicated in some haemolytic anaemias as well as in haemochromatosis

E is effective by the oral route for chronic iron overload

30.7 Vitamin B$_{12}$

A stores in the body are enough to last for six weeks

B is normally absorbed by the terminal ileum

C therapy for pernicious anaemia may be initially complicated by severe hypokalaemia

D is sensible trial therapy in undiagnosed anaemias

E may be used in large doses by mouth where injections are impracticable

30.8 Folic acid

A prevents neural tube defect in pregnancies subsequent to an affected birth

B alone is adequate treatment for megaloblastic anaemia

C is active only when converted to tetrahydrofolic acid

D is not present in green vegetables other than spinach

E should not be used routinely in pregnancy for fear of masking co-existent pernicious anaemia

30.9 The following statements about haemopoietic growth factors are correct:

A Epoetin is effective treatment for the anaemia of chronic renal failure

B Use of epoetin may lead to hypertension

C Epoetin use may cause arteriovenous shunts to thrombose

D Filgrastim is used to treat bone marrow depression by cytotoxic drugs

E Molgramostim has a narrower spectrum of activity than filgrastim

31 Neoplastic disease and immunosuppression

31.1 **In the chemotherapy of malignant disease the following statements are historically correct:**

A The first attempt to control cancer by means other than surgery was not made until the end of the nineteenth century

B Observation that oophorectomy prolonged lactation in cows led to the suggestion that some cases of breast cancer are dependent on ovarian function

C Regression of prostatic cancer due to oestrogens was observed 46 years later

D Depression of haemopoiesis by sulphur mustards (the precursors of nitrogen mustards) was observed when they were used as chemical weapons in the 1914–18 World War

E Nitrogen mustards had to be first tested for therapeutic effect on humans since no satisfactory animal model was available

31.2 **Success of chemotherapy in malignant disease depends on**

A the sensitivity of malignant cells to drugs
B the size of the tumour
C the number of cells dividing at any one time
D the endocrine environment of the malignant cell
E the rate of recovery of normal tissues from the effects of treatment

31.3 Cancer cells

A have less differentiated morphology than the tissue of origin

B divide more rapidly than the cells in any normal organ

C exhibit circadian rhythms in proliferation

D are generally most sensitive to drugs when they are in a resting phase

E are not subject to the normal feedback mechanism which restricts cell multiplication

31.4 Factors which tend to make an ageing cancer less susceptible to drugs include

A decrease in the number of cells actively dividing

B increased cell cycle (division) time

C a defective vascular supply

D increased cell death within the tumour

E overcrowding of cells, denying access to drugs

31.5 The following statements on principles of chemotherapy in cancer are correct:

A A given dose of drug kills a constant number of cells, however many are present

B Intermittent combination chemotherapy depends partly on selecting drugs that act at the same phases of the growth cycle

C Part of the reasoning underlying intermittent chemotherapy is to allow suppressed immunological mechanisms to recover

D Inadequate initial therapy is the usual reason for failure to control cancers that are curable by chemotherapy

E Multiple drug resistance may be due to a membrane efflux pump developed as a protective mechanism against environmental toxins

31.6 **In planning intermittent combination therapy**

A vincristine is used to synchronise active cell cycles
B most regimens have been devised on a basis of common-sense empiricism
C intervals between courses of drugs should be at least two months
D cycle-specific agents are given before those that are cycle-non-specific
E overlap of toxicities between the drugs chosen is of little importance

31.7 **Adverse effects of anticancer drugs include**

A depression of both antibody and cell-mediated immunity
B irreversible alopecia
C reproductive sterility
D urate nephropathy
E a temporary mutagenic effect on gonadal cells

31.8 **Adverse effects of anticancer drugs include**

A occurrence of second cancer five years or more after treatment
B risk to pregnant health staff from handling drugs
C opportunistic infection with protozoon organisms, e.g. *Pneumocystis carinii*
D vomiting which is best managed by a drug combination
E teratogenicity

31.9 **The following statements about hormone-dependent cancer are correct:**

A Adrenocortical hormones, though useful for complications, have no direct action on the cancer itself
B Prostate cancer is androgen-dependent
C Treatment of prostate cancer with a gonadotrophin analogue may transiently exacerbate bone pain
D About 60% of patients with oestrogen-receptor positive breast cancer respond to hormonal manipulation
E In breast cancer tamoxifen is the adjuvant therapy of choice for postmenopausal women who have disease in the lymph nodes

31.10 **The following statements about cytotoxic agents are correct:**

A Alkylating agents interfere with normal DNA synthesis
B Methotrexate competitively inhibits dihydrofolate reductase
C Folinic acid (calcium leucovorin) terminates the action of methotrexate
D Active tubular secretion of methotrexate is blocked by salicylate (from aspirin) with increased risk of toxicity
E Azathioprine acts by depriving cells of essential metabolites

31.11 **In the field of cytotoxic agents**

A radiophosphorus is the treatment of choice for polycythaemia vera in older patients
B daunorubicin use may cause cardiomyopathy
C vincristine causes cell cycle arrest in mitosis
D antibiotics such as bleomycin interfere with DNA/RNA synthesis
E it is now generally agreed that laetrile can relieve pain and prolong survival

31.12 One of the first choice drugs for

A chronic lymphocytic leukaemia is chlorambucil
B oesophageal cancer is cisplatin
C brain cancer is procarbazine
D ovary cancer is cisplatin
E choriocarcinoma is actinomycin D

31.13 In immunosuppressive therapy

A cyclosporin selectively inhibits multiplication of the immunocompetent T-lymphocyte
B cyclosporin may cause hypertension
C development of severe chickenpox is a hazard
D carcinogenicity is not a long-term hazard
E antilymphocytic globulin does not induce allergy

31.14 The following statements about immunomodulation and biological therapy for cancer are correct:

A Aldesleukin (interleukin-2) is used to treat metastases in renal cell cancer
B Interferon alfa may be used for hairy cell leukaemia
C During immunosuppression, response to living vaccines, e.g. some polio vaccines, may cause serious generalised disease
D During immunosuppression, a normal response to nonliving antigens, e.g. tetanus, may be expected
E Human gammaglobulin has no place in protecting patients taking immunosuppressive drugs

32 Stomach and oesophagus

32.1   Histamine H$_2$-receptor antagonists

- A   increase the healing rate of peptic ulcers
- B   should not be used to prevent recurrent peptic ulcers
- C   do not benefit reflux oesophagitis
- D   do not relieve the symptoms of malignant gastric ulcer
- E   are used to prevent bleeding from gastric erosions complicating the stress of serious conditions, e.g. burns

32.2   Cimetidine

- A   inhibits hepatic metabolism of other drugs
- B   inhibits gastric secretion stimulated by caffeine
- C   may be of value for chronic pancreatic insufficiency
- D   treatment approximately doubles the spontaneous healing rate of gastric ulcer
- E   may cause gynaecomastia

32.3   In the treatment of peptic ulcer the following statements are correct:

- A   Ranitidine reduces gastric acid less effectively than does cimetidine
- B   Pirenzepine reduces gastric acid through selective antimuscarinic action
- C   Long-term suppression of gastric secretion leads to the development of gastric cancer
- D   Proton pump inhibitors such as omeprazole antagonise all stimulants of gastric secretion
- E   There is no need to adjust the dose of phenytoin for a patient who starts treatment with omeprazole

32.4   The following statements about antacids are correct:

A   Metabolic alkalosis is more likely to occur with sodium bicarbonate than with other antacids

B   Magnesium salts cause diarrhoea

C   Long-term use of calcium-containing antacids should be avoided since they may produce renal damage

D   Aluminium hydroxide is the antacid of choice for patients in renal failure

E   Certain antacids are likely to produce oedema in patients with cardiac disease

32.5   The following statements about drugs and mucosal resistance are correct:

A   Bismuth chelate acts only by coating the base of a peptic ulcer

B   Bismuth chelate is the preferred agent to heal peptic ulcers in patients with impaired renal function

C   Sucralfate has a potent acid-neutralising capacity

D   Eradication of *Helicobacter pylori* protects against relapse of duodenal ulcer

E   *Helicobacter pylori* is sensitive to amoxicillin

32.6   The following statements about treatment of peptic ulcer are correct:

A   Misoprostol prevents the formation of gastric ulcer in patients taking nonsteroidal anti-inflammatory drugs

B   Misoprostol is the preferred treatment for gastric ulcer in pregnant women

C   Ulcers that are difficult to heal with a histamine H_2-receptor blocker may respond to omeprazole

D   Relapse of duodenal ulcer may be prevented by a single dose of a histamine H_2-receptor blocker taken nightly

E   Concurrent use of antacids with histamine H_2-receptor blocker is contraindicated

32.7 **The following statements about vomiting and antiemetic drugs are correct:**

A   Antiemetic agents that act on the vomiting centre allay vomiting from any cause

B   The chemoreceptor trigger zone (CTZ) is rich in dopamine D_2-receptors

C   Antiemetics that act on the vomiting centre are predominantly antimuscarinic

D   Metoclopramide acts by blockade of muscarinic receptors

E   Metoclopramide may cause dystonic reactions

32.8 **The following statements about antiemetic drugs are correct:**

A   Domperidone blocks dopamine D_2-receptors in the chemoreceptor trigger zone and upper gut

B   Domperidone commonly causes dystonic reactions

C   Ondansetron is ineffective against vomiting induced by cytotoxic agents

D   Ondansetron is a selective $5\text{-}HT_3$-receptor antagonist

E   Cisapride has a strong sedative effect

32.9 **The following statements about vomiting are correct:**

A   Motion sickness responds well to drugs with antimuscarinic actions

B   Drug-induced vomiting responds well to metoclopramide

C   The cytotoxic drug cisplatin frequently causes vomiting

D   Postoperative vomiting responds to haloperidol

E   Dexamethasone is effective treatment for cytotoxic drug-induced vomiting

33 Intestines

33.1 **The following statements about bulk laxatives are correct:**

A They act by reducing the volume and raising the viscosity of bowel contents

B Bran may cause intestinal obstruction if taken with too little fluid

C Over-use of bran may cause heartburn

D Dietary fibre comprises the cell walls and supporting structures of vegetables and fruits

E Soluble fibre may be used to improve glycaemic control in diabetics

33.2 **The following statements about laxatives are correct:**

A Lactulose is an osmotic laxative

B The fermentation to acids of lactulose (in the colon) benefits hepatic encephalopathy

C Osmotic laxatives are all well-absorbed from the colon

D Methylcellulose takes up water to form a colloid 25 times its original volume

E Docusate sodium softens hard faeces

33.3 **The following statements about stimulant laxatives are correct:**

A   Use of bisacodyl is severely limited by adverse effects
B   Some anthraquinone preparations cause the urine to turn red
C   Long-term use of preparations containing danthron is acceptable
D   Oxyphenisatin is safe for long-term use
E   Prolonged use of anthraquinone group laxatives may lead to melanosis coli

33.4 **The following statements about laxative use and constipation are correct:**

A   Senna is acceptable for use in pregnancy
B   Long-term use of stimulant laxatives may damage the myenteric pathways of the colon
C   Stimulant purgatives are appropriate therapy to get rid of hardened faeces in the rectum
D   When treating intractable pain with an opioid, a laxative should be prescribed with the analgesic
E   Calcium channel blockers may cause constipation

33.5 **Oral rehydration therapy of acute diarrhoea**

A   is effectively achieved by a solution containing glucose, sodium, chloride, potassium and bicarbonate
B   alone is sufficient to treat most episodes of watery diarrhoea
C   may usefully utilise carbohydrate from a variety of sources
D   is not well achieved by commercial soft drinks because of their low sodium content
E   should always be accompanied by an antimotility drug in controlling severe diarrhoea in young children

33.6   In the treatment of diarrhoea

A   kaolin has marginal therapeutic efficacy
B   opioid drugs delay passage of gut contents by reducing peristalsis and increasing segmentation
C   diphenoxylate may cause severe respiratory depression if taken in overdose
D   loperamide has a high potential for abuse
E   in patients with colostomy, ispaghula may provide benefit

33.7   In treatment of inflammatory bowel disease

A   hydrocortisone i.v. should be used for a severe attack of ulcerative colitis
B   prednisolone by mouth and a 5-aminosalicylic acid agent should be used for a mild attack of ulcerative colitis
C   metronidazole may improve perianal Crohn's disease
D   azathioprine should not be used in Crohn's disease
E   diarrhoea due to faecal loading should be treated with a laxative

33.8   Of the 5-aminosalicylic acid compounds

A   sulphasalazine causes reversible infertility in men
B   sulphasalazine causes more adverse effects than mesalazine
C   mesalazine acts in the small intestine
D   mesalazine is effective for maintaining remission of ulcerative colitis
E   olsalazine contains a sulphonamide component

34 Liver, biliary tract, pancreas

34.1 **Hepatic injury due to**
A paracetamol is not dose-dependent
B tetracyclines occurs at high doses
C halothane is dose-related
D chlorpromazine is cholestatic
E rifampicin only occurs after several months of treatment

34.2 **The following statements about drugs and the liver are correct:**
A Amiodarone may cause cirrhosis
B Oral contraceptive use for more than 5 years may cause benign hepatic tumours
C Fibrosis due to methotrexate can be minimised by using small daily doses
D Isoniazid may cause chronic active hepatitis
E Fusidic acid may cause jaundice

34.3 **In a patient with cirrhosis of the liver**
A drugs normally subject to high hepatic first-pass metabolism have a low systemic availability
B drugs normally subject to low hepatic first-pass metabolism exhibit prolongation of $t\frac{1}{2}$
C a nonsteroidal anti-inflammatory drug is more likely to cause sodium retention
D morphine is safe in normal doses
E sensitivity to warfarin is decreased

34.4 The following statements about prescribing for patients with liver disease are correct:

A The initial dose of nifedipine should be small
B Antacids containing sodium may cause fluid retention
C A potassium-sparing drug should be included in a diuretic regimen
D MAO inhibitors are less hazardous than tricyclic antidepressants
E Antimicrobials normally eliminated by the kidney are safe in normal doses

34.5 In a patient with gallstones

A ursodeoxycholic acid can be expected to dissolve calcified stones
B chenodeoxycholic acid is the preferred treatment for pregnant women
C ursodeoxycholic acid is less likely to cause diarrhoea than chenodeoxycholic acid
D drug treatment is likely to require 24 months to be effective
E cholestyramine is only indicated to relieve pruritus if bile duct obstruction is complete

35 Adrenal corticosteroids, antagonists, corticotrophin

35.1 **The naturally-occurring physiologically important secretions of the adrenal cortex include**

A   cortisone
B   hydrocortisone
C   prednisolone
D   aldosterone
E   androgens

35.2 **The following statements about natural corticotrophin are correct:**

A   It is a polypeptide consisting of 39 amino acids
B   All its biological effect requires all the amino acids
C   Its immunological antigenic activity resides in the final 15 aminoacids
D   It has a plasma $t\frac{1}{2}$ of 3 hours
E   The response of the adrenal cortex to a rise in plasma corticotrophin begins after 30 minutes

35.3 **Natural corticotrophin**

A   is active when taken by mouth
B   is the major controlling factor in hydrocortisone production by the adrenal cortex
C   is the major controlling factor in aldosterone production by the adrenal cortex
D   is a preferred treatment for Addison's disease (primary adrenocortical insufficiency)
E   is a preferred treatment for secondary adrenocortical insufficiency (hypopituitarism)

35.4 Tetracosactrin

A is a synthetic polypeptide
B has an amino acid structure identical with natural corticotrophin
C is more liable to induce immunological adverse reactions (allergy) than is corticotrophin obtained from animals
D has a plasma $t\frac{1}{2}$ much longer than natural corticotrophin
E is active when taken by mouth

35.5 The following corticosteroids are best avoided because they require metabolic conversion to become biologically active:

A Hydrocortisone
B Cortisone
C Prednisone
D Prednisolone
E Methylprednisolone

35.6 The following statements about adrenocortical steroids are correct:

A Mineralocorticoid actions principally enhance sodium excretion and potassium retention
B Glucocorticoid actions principally affect metabolism of carbohydrate, protein and fat
C Glucocorticoid actions include suppression of inflammation and of immune responses
D Systemic administration of substantial doses induces suppression of the hypothalamic-pituitary-adrenocortical system via a feedback mechanism
E Lymphoid tissue is reduced

35.7 **The following substances have largely or exclusively mineralocorticoid actions:**

A Dexamethasone
B Hydrocortisone
C Fludrocortisone
D Prednisolone
E Spironolactone

35.8 **An adrenal cortex suppressed by administration of a high therapeutic dose of adrenocortical steroid**

A continues to secrete androgen
B continues to secrete aldosterone
C will recover independently of hypothalamic-pituitary function
D puts the patient at hazard due to intercurrent disease
E puts patients at hazard if they lose their tablets

35.9 **The following statements about the quantitative aspects of adrenocortical steroid function and therapy are correct:**

A The normal daily secretion of hydrocortisone is 10–30 mg which is equivalent to prednisolone 2.5–7.5 mg
B Prednisolone 5 mg administered regularly as a late evening dose will suppress the normal early morning rise in plasma cortisol
C High doses (pharmacotherapy) of corticosteroid induce clinically important suppression of the hypothalamic-pituitary-adrenocortical axis within one week
D Recovery of hypothalamic-pituitary-adrenocortical function is complete one week after withdrawal of a suppressive dose of corticosteroid
E When prednisolone is administered for more than a month, the risk of serious adverse effects is poorly predicted by the dose and duration of prescribing

35.10 Adrenocortical steroids are of established vallue when used

A as replacement therapy in adrenocortical insufficiency
B for hypercalcaemia of sarcoidosis
C in myasthenia gravis
D to suppress immunological inflammation
E to suppress the rejection of transplanted organs

35.11 The following choices of corticosteroid are appropriate:

A Prednisone for replacement therapy
B Beclomethasone for inhalation in asthma
C Cortisone for topical skin use
D Prednisolone for anti-inflammation
E Dexamethasone for reduction of intracranial pressure

35.12 The following statements about adrenocortical steroid therapy are correct:

A Atrophy of the adrenal cortex in long-term treatment is due to a direct effect on the hypothalamus
B During withdrawal, adrenocortical hormone should be substituted to prevent symptoms of hypoadrenalism
C Therapy should be stopped immediately an adverse effect appears
D Triamcinolone has negligible sodium retaining effect
E Dexamethasone has low anti-inflammatory effect

35.13 Replacement therapy with corticosteroid

A is best conducted with hydrocortisone because it has both mineralocorticoid and glucocorticoid effects
B is devised to mimic the pattern of natural hormone secretion during day and night
C is conducted at higher doses than pharmacotherapy
D may be undertaken with corticotrophin
E usually includes a small dose of fludrocortisone

35.14 In long-term corticosteroid pharmacotherapy for anti-inflammatory effect

A beclomethasone is especially useful by inhalation in asthma as the inevitable 90% which is swallowed is extensively metabolised by the liver
B triamcinolone is liable to cause muscle wasting
C prednisolone is preferable to hydrocortisone because prednisolone has selective glucocorticoid actions
D fluorinated compounds, e.g. triamcinolone, are best avoided in pregnant women as they are teratogenic in animals
E an injection of corticotrophin should be given regularly to prevent cortical atrophy

35.15 Indications for courses of adrenocortical steroids include

A sarcoidosis
B Addison's disease
C acute gout
D nephrotic syndrome
E hay fever

35.16 Long-term adrenocortical steroid therapy carries an extra risk of adverse effects in patients giving a history of

A mental disorder
B peptic ulcer
C hypertension
D tuberculosis
E diabetes mellitus

35.17 Active immunisation of patients taking long-term corticosteroid pharmacotherapy (for suppression of inflammation or immune responses)

A should never be attempted in children
B is hazardous with a killed vaccine
C is hazardous with a live vaccine
D is hazardous with a toxoid vaccine
E may be ineffective if the dose of corticosteroid is high

35.18 **If patients on long-term corticosteroid therapy (whether for replacement or pharmacotherapy) develop an intercurrent illness, they should**

A omit the next dose
B double their next dose and inform their doctor
C take large doses of oral potassium
D save a specimen of urine for the doctor to test
E be admitted to hospital for parenteral hydrocortisone

35.19 **Precautions to be taken during high dose long-term corticosteroid pharmacotherapy include**

A regular weighing
B regular blood pressure measurement
C a regular urine test for glucose
D carrying a special card recording the details of treatment
E paying serious attention to any illness, however slight

35.20 **Adverse effects of long-term corticosteroid pharmacotherapy include**

A osteoporosis
B hypertension
C muscle wasting
D deficient blood coagulation
E alopecia

35.21 **A patient who has taken corticosteroid for a long time may develop**

A psychotic reaction
B increased growth in children
C menstrual disorders
D major skin damage after quite minor injury
E raised intracranial pressure

35.22 Long-term corticosteroid pharmacotherapy may lead to

A avascular necrosis of bone
B serious delayed tissue healing after surgery
C increased severity of infections
D masking of infections, which may produce atypical clinical features
E activation of dormant infections

35.23 The following statements about withdrawing adrenocorticosteroid pharmacotherapy that has lasted for many weeks are correct:

A The patient is at risk of acute adrenal insufficiency because the adrenal cortex has atrophied
B The longer the duration of therapy, the slower must be the withdrawal
C Withdrawal of prednisolone at the rate of 1 mg per day per month is appropriate
D If a patient cannot take the dose orally there should be no hesitation in using an injectable (i.m.) preparation
E If a patient requires surgery during, or even one year after withdrawal, a careful scheme of added corticosteroid administration is required

35.24 In pregnancy

A corticosteroid pharmacotherapy is generally well tolerated by mother and fetus
B fluorinated corticosteroids carry teratogenic hazard, even if applied to the skin
C hypoadrenal patients on replacement therapy require no special management
D labour is managed like major surgery
E the effects of high dose corticosteroid pharmacotherapy to the mother may not affect the child until shortly after birth

35.25 The following statements about adrenocortical hormone synthesis and function are correct:

A Spironolactone is a competitive antagonist of aldosterone

B Metyrapone blocks corticosteroid receptors

C Formestane inhibits the conversion of androgens to oestrogens and is used to treat some patients with breast cancer

D Metyrapone can be used as a test for the capacity of the hypothalamic-pituitary axis to produce corticotrophin

E Trilostane interferes with enzymatic synthesis of hydrocortisone and of aldosterone

36 Diabetes mellitus, insulin, oral antidiabetes agents

36.1 Insulin

A output by the pancreas is 30–40 units daily
B antibodies develop in all patients treated with animal insulins
C activity does not differ as between human and animal forms
D is stored in the liver
E is a polypeptide

36.2 Insulin causes

A reduction of hepatic output of glucose
B reduction of protein synthesis
C enhanced transit of potassium into cells
D increased glucose uptake in peripheral tissues
E down-regulation of insulin receptors when its concentration is high, a factor in the insulin resistance of obese diabetics

36.3 When insulin is injected

A about half the dose can be recovered from the urine
B s.c. or i.v. the time-course of its action is similar
C and hypoglycaemia results, corticotrophin is released from the pituitary
D the intravenous route is preferred in severe ketoacidosis
E subcutaneous lipoatrophy is common with the human variety

36.4   Soluble insulin

A   is presented as an aqueous solution adjusted to pH 7.0
B   if infused in a saline drip is subject to substantial loss as a result of binding to the tubing
C   has a $t\frac{1}{2}$ of 5 minutes when given intravenously
D   is particularly useful for balancing patients who have heavy glycosuria before breakfast (Somogyi effect)
E   is the only insulin preparation suitable for intravenous use

36.5   In the confusing terminology surrounding insulin formulations

A   soluble and neutral insulin are the same
B   isophane insulin is the only approved name for suspensions of insulin with protamine
C   mixed insulins are not the same as biphasic insulins
D   biphasic insulins provide a range of soluble insulin concentrations between 10% and 50% of the total insulin concentration
E   mixed insulin suspension is the approved name for proprietary mixtures of crystalline and amorphous zinc suspension

36.6   A hypoglycaemic attack

A   should always be treated by giving sugar (sucrose or glucose) in the first instance
B   which does not respond to glucose within 30 minutes suggests that dexamethasone may be useful as the patient may have cerebral oedema
C   if severe may cause permanent damage to the central nervous system
D   should be treated by glucagon injections only if there has been no response one hour after intravenous glucose
E   may be caused by a biguanide used alone

36.7 The following statements about oral hypoglycaemic drugs are correct:

A Biguanides are effective even in the absence of insulin
B Sulphonylureas act by stimulating the β-islet cells of the pancreas
C Chlorpropamide is safer than gliclazide in patients with poor renal function
D Lactic acidosis does not occur with metformin
E Glibenclamide must be taken three times a day

36.8 In the treatment of diabetes it is generally accepted that

A patients should reduce their insulin dosage if they develop intercurrent illness
B weight loss is associated with an increase in the number of insulin receptors, and response to insulin
C a fasting blood glucose of <6 mmol/l and a 2-hour postprandial glucose of <9 mmol/l represents good control
D once a patient has been stabilised on an oral hypoglycaemic drug, close supervision is no longer needed
E good control of blood sugar in insulin dependent diabetes mellitus (IDDM) reduces the incidence of neuropathy and nephropathy

36.9 In a pregnant diabetic patient

A oral hypoglycaemic agents are preferable to insulin
B insulin requirements are lower immediately after delivery and during the first 6 weeks of lactation
C the renal threshold for glucose rises
D maternal hyperglycaemia leads to fetal islet cell hyperplasia
E all treatment for diabetes should be stopped during labour

36.10 Drugs which can disturb the control of a diabetic patient include

A   monoamine oxidase inhibitors
B   β-adrenoceptor blockers
C   cimetidine
D   thiazide diuretics
E   combined oral contraceptives

36.11 In diabetic ketoacidosis

A   substantial body deficit of potassium is present
B   fluid replacement is the first priority
C   insulin is best given by continuous low-dose i.v. infusion
D   insulin corrects acidosis
E   bicarbonate should be administered when the arterial pH is <7.0

36.12 In a diabetic undergoing major surgery

A   a high blood glucose concentration, even for a short time, is particularly dangerous
B   insulin is indicated even if there has been previous good control by oral hypoglycaemic drugs
C   insulin requirements are likely to be higher as a result of operation
D   glucose by mouth should be given one hour preoperatively
E   ketoacidosis should be controlled, if possible, in all cases before operation, even in a surgical emergency

36.13 In the treatment of non-insulin dependent diabetes mellitus (NIDDM)

A   in an obese patient, the drug of choice is metformin
B   insulin may be required for glycaemic control
C   acarbose reduces carbohydrate absorption by inhibiting α-glucosidase in the gut
D   chlorpropamide is preferred for elderly patients
E   oral hypoglycaemic agents can successfully be withdrawn from about 30% of patients after a few months

36.14 **The following statements about the treatment of diabetes are correct:**

A Insulin resistance may be treated by immunosuppression

B Insulin resistance may be inherited

C Insulin emp, pyr, and prb indicate the sources from which insulin is derived

D Awareness of hypoglycaemia may be reduced when human insulin is taken

E Monocomponent porcine insulin is more immunogenic than bovine insulin

37 Thyroid hormones, antithyroid drugs

37.1 Thyroid hormone

A consists of L-thyroxine (T_4) and liothyronine (T_3)
B exerts its effect chiefly through T_3 to which T_4 is converted
C is 99.9% bound to plasma protein
D acts on specific nuclear receptors
E is stored in the gland as thyroglobulin

37.2 Treatment with thyroxine

A can reduce the size of puberty goitre
B is accepted therapy for simple obesity
C requires that tablets be taken three times per day
D for hypothyroidism should be monitored by the plasma TSH concentration
E for hypothyroidism during pregnancy may necessitate an increase in dose

37.3 The following statements about thyroid hormone treatment are correct:

A Liothyronine finds its main use in hypothyroid coma
B A dose of liothyronine gives maximum effect in about 24 h and passes off over 48 h
C Hydrocortisone may also be necessary when prolonged hypothyroidism is treated
D Slight overtreatment may cause atrial fibrillation in patients over 60 years
E Overtreatment causes exophthalmos

37.4   Iodine or iodide

A   in radiographic contrast media may cause fatal anaphylaxis
B   is an effective antiseptic
C   given preoperatively makes thyroidectomy easier and safe
D   in small amounts is useful in cough medicines
E   can cause goitre

37.5   The following statements about thiourea derivatives are correct:

A   They inhibit the coupling of iodotyrosine to form T_4 and T_3
B   They are not goitrogenic
C   Carbimazole cannot be expected to cause any clinical improvement in less than a month
D   Normal doses should be used in pregnancy as they do not cross the placenta
E   Their effect may be monitored by the ankle reflex time

37.6   When a β-adrenoceptor blocker is used in the treatment of hyperthyroidism

A   small doses relieve symptoms but not the overproduction of thyroxine
B   propranolol does not have a role if radioiodine is being used
C   a $β_1$-selective agent should be used
D   timolol eyedrops may improve ocular symptoms
E   the dose can be monitored by the heart rate

37.7 The following statements about the use of radioiodine (^{131}I) are correct:

A Most hyperthyroid patients treated with radioiodine are likely to need treatment for hypothyroidism eventually
B The effect is maximal in 3 weeks
C Women of child-bearing age should be advised not to get pregnant for 6 months after treatment
D There is no increased risk of leukaemia even after the high doses needed for treatment of thyroid carcinoma
E Low dose will suffice to treat a single hyperfunctioning 'hot' nodule

37.8 The following statements about radioiodine are correct:

A Radioiodine treatment for hyperthyroidism is likely to damage the parathyroid glands
B Pregnant women may be treated with radioiodine as it does not cross the placenta
C Overdose of radioiodine should be treated by large doses of sodium or potassium iodide
D ^{131}I has a physical (radioactive) $t_{\frac{1}{2}}$ of 8 days
E Radioiodine treatment of thyroid cancer carries a late risk of leukaemia

37.9 Hypothyroidism may be caused by

A resorcinol
B amiodarone
C lithium
D atenolol
E digoxin

38 Hypothalamic, pituitary and sex hormones

38.1 Among the anterior pituitary hormones

A naturally occurring human growth hormone is identical to the recombinant molecules now preferred for therapeutic uses

B the plasma half-life of corticotrophin is 10 minutes

C prolactin is secreted only by women

D human chorionic gonadotrophin (HCG) induces progesterone production in the corpus luteum

E HCG is valueless for cryptorchidism in prepubertal males

38.2 In infertility

A in a hypopituitary woman, treatment with follicle stimulating hormone (FSH) is required to achieve ovulation

B of non-hypopituitary anovular origin, blockade of hypothalamic oestrogen receptors may cause ovulation

C clomiphene treatment carries an increased risk of multiple pregnancy

D tamoxifen has a part to play in the treatment of both female and male infertility

E testosterone is the hormone of choice in the treatment of male infertility

38.3 Vasopressin

A increases water reabsorption in the renal collecting duct

B secretion is stimulated by nicotine

C deficiency may occur in hypopituitarism

D is a useful drug to raise the blood pressure

E may cause angina through coronary artery vasoconstriction

38.4 In diabetes insipidus

A thiazide diuretics sometimes have an antidiuretic effect
B glibenclamide may produce clinical improvement
C demeclocycline is beneficial
D lithium is beneficial
E desmopressin is the treatment of choice

38.5 The syndrome of inappropriate antidiuretic hormone secretion (SIADH)

A is caused only by oat-cell lung cancer
B may be treated by fluid restriction and fludrocortisone
C when acute should be treated with infusion of hypertonic saline
D may be usefully treated by demeclocycline
E is unaffected by chemotherapy to a causal tumour

38.6 Oxytocin

A is used to prevent premature labour
B can be used to enhance milk ejection from the breast
C obtained from the posterior pituitary gland is safer than the synthetic product (Syntocinon)
D treatment mimics normal uterine activity in labour
E use may lead to water intoxication

38.7 Testosterone

A is necessary for spermatogenesis as well as for growth of the sexual apparatus
B is used to treat sterility in primary hypogonadism
C is antagonised by cyproterone
D may be useful in the prevention of osteoporosis in males
E slows the rate of closure of epiphyses of bone

38.8 Cyproterone

A has affinity for androgen receptors both in peripheral target organs and in the central nervous system
B is a derivative of progesterone
C causes irreversible reduction of spermatogenesis in males
D is used in female hirsutism
E exacerbates acne

38.9 When treated with a protein anabolic agent

A adult males run a substantial risk of hypermasculinisation
B patients with advanced malignant disease may feel better
C the itching of jaundice may lessen
D men with established osteoporosis can be expected to improve
E the unwanted catabolic effects of adrenocortical hormones are reduced

38.10 The following statements about oestrogens are correct:

A The vagina is more sensitive to oestrogens than is the endometrium
B They are as effective as androgens in promoting closure of epiphyses
C Stilboestrol administered to mothers caused vaginal adenocarcinoma in their daughters
D Their use in postmenopausal hormone replacement therapy (HRT) prevents osteoporosis
E Patients with senile vaginitis may use oestrogen pessaries without risk of systemic effects

38.11 In oestrogen replacement therapy

A 'unopposed' treatment, i.e. without added progestogen, increases risk of endometrial carcinoma
B continuous treatment is preferable to interrupted courses
C risk of breast cancer is reduced
D cyclical use is essential in hysterectomised women
E adding progestogen, for menopausal symptoms, can be regarded as adequate for hormonal contraception

38.12 Oestrogen treatment

A may be used to reduce sexual urge in men
B may precipitate migraine
C may benefit acne
D may lead to thromboembolism
E inhibits lactation by the same mechanism as does bromocriptine

38.13 The following statements about progesterone or its derivatives are correct:

A Progesterone is necessary for implantation of the ovum
B Prolonged use may cause blood pressure to rise
C Administration of gestodene to the mother can virilise a female fetus
D Danazol is used to treat endometriosis
E Mifepristone is effective treatment for threatened abortion

38.14 In the control of conception

A gonadorelin (LH/FSH/RH), used continuously, suppresses spermatogenesis by down-regulation of its receptors
B permanent damage to fertility after stopping hormonal contraception is very rare
C vaginal preparations such as nonoxinol are highly reliable if properly used
D the safe period after a missed dose depends on the amount of oestrogen in the formulation used
E postcoital contraception with an oestrogen-progesterone combined preparation is effective up to 72 hours after exposure

38.15 The effects of oral contraception with a mixture of oestrogen and progestogen include

A decreased viscosity of cervical mucus
B a substantial risk of harming an undiagnosed pregnancy
C decreased glucose tolerance
D liability to premenstrual tension
E a reduced risk of carcinoma of the ovary

38.16 Oral oestrogen/progestogen contraceptives

A may precipitate migraine
B reduce the risk of cardiovascular complications in smokers
C are suitable for a woman with breast cancer
D do not increase the risk of gallbladder disease
E should be withdrawn 4 weeks before major elective surgery

38.17 In the treatment of menstruation and its disorders

A the premenstrual tension syndrome is well controlled by bromocriptine
B dysmenorrhoea is usefully treated by inhibitors of prostaglandin synthesis
C cyclical breast pain may respond to gamolenic acid
D menorrhagia may be reduced by norethisterone
E endometriosis responds best to an oestrogen-progesterone oral contraceptive administered for about 9 months

38.18 The following statements about ergot derivatives are correct:

A Ergometrine is preferred for the prevention and treatment of postpartum haemorrhage
B Oxytocin is preferred for induction of labour
C Ergotamine is an α-adrenoceptor agonist
D Cabergoline suppresses prolactin secretion
E Ergometrine can cause severe hypertension

38.19 The following statements about drugs and the uterus are correct:

A β_2-adrenoceptor agonists used during labour may lead to severe left ventricular failure

B β_2-adrenoceptor agonists are used to induce labour

C Dinoprost (prostaglandin $F_2\alpha$) is effective for preventing premature labour

D Carboprost (a prostaglandin $F_2\alpha$ analogue) is effective for postpartum haemorrhage

E Gemeprost (a prostaglandin E_1 analogue) is used to induce abortion

38.20 The following drugs may cause hyperprolactinaemia:

A Metoclopramide

B Apomorphine

C Bromocriptine

D Chlorpromazine

E Methyldopa

39 Vitamins, calcium, bone

39.1 Vitamin A

- A as isotretinoin may be used to prevent squamous cell carcinomas of the head and neck
- B in the form of tretinoin benefits acne
- C in overdose causes painful swelling on long bones
- D in above physiological amounts is teratogenic in humans
- E deficiency causes epithelial keratosis

39.2 The following statements about the B group of vitamins are correct:

- A Thiamine (B_1) is used to treat Wernicke-Korsakoff psychosis
- B Pyridoxine (B_6) is used in the treatment of homocystinuria
- C Pyridoxine deficiency may be induced by isoniazid
- D Overdose of pyridoxine causes peripheral neuropathy
- E Nicotinic acid (B_7) may cause flushing

39.3 Vitamin C (ascorbic acid)

- A may be used to treat methaemoglobinaemia
- B taken in high dose may lead to the formation of urinary tract oxalate stones
- C decreases absorption of iron from the intestine
- D given i.v. may precipitate haemolysis in patients with glucose-6-phosphate dehydrogenase deficiency
- E is commonly used to acidify urine as part of the treatment of poisoning

39.4 Methaemoglobinaemia

A impairs the oxygen carrying capacity of the blood
B may be due to treatment with sulphonamides
C may be due to treatment with primaquine
D may be caused by nitrates
E is more effectively treated with ascorbic acid than methylene blue

39.5 The following statements about vitamin D preparations are correct:

A Calcitriol is the least active natural form
B Alfacalcidol is indicated for vitamin D therapy needed for a patient with renal failure
C Alfacalcidol has a slow onset of action
D Patients treated with phenytoin may require vitamin D
E Overdose of vitamin D may lead to renal failure

39.6 The following statements about plasma and urinary calcium are correct:

A Acute hypocalcaemia should be treated with rapid injection of calcium gluconate
B A plasma calcium concentration of 3.0 mmol/l does not call for urgent treatment
C Cellulose phosphate by mouth is used to treat chronic hypercalcaemia
D A thiazide diuretic is useful treatment for patients who form urinary calcium stones
E Trisodium edetate i.v. is valuable treatment for chronic hypercalcaemia

39.7 Acute hypercalcaemia is benefited by

A controlled rehydration
B frusemide
C dialysis
D plicamycin (mithramycin) if the cause is cancer
E oral phosphate

39.8   Calcitonin

A   is a steroid hormone
B   is produced in the thymus remnant
C   enhances the rate of bone turnover
D   is used to control bone pain in Paget's disease of bone
E   is used to control hypercalcaemia

39.9   In osteoporosis

A   due to gonadal deficiency, a progestogen arrests the process by increasing bone formation
B   due to gonadal deficiency, oestrogen arrests the process by reducing bone absorption
C   sudden cessation of oestrogen treatment leads to enhanced bone loss
D   biphosphonates with calcium reduce the incidence of vertebral fracture
E   may be treated more effectively with sodium fluoride than with biphosphonates

39.10   The following statements about paget's disease of bone and vitamin E are correct:

A   Biphosphonates are the treatment of choice for Paget's disease
B   Paget's disease is characterised by abnormally slow bone turnover
C   Vitamin E deficiency is associated with spinocerebellar degeneration
D   Vitamin E may act principally as a scavenger of free radicals produced by normal intermediary metabolism
E   Vitamin E may have a role in the treatment of ischaemic heart disease

39.11   The pain of Paget's disease of bone may be relieved by

A   improving the blood supply with tocopherols
B   inhibiting bone resorption with calcitonin
C   inhibiting crystal formation with biphosphonate
D   inhibiting osteoclasts with a cytotoxic agent
E   increasing osteocyte activity with parathormone

Answers

Question	Answer
1	BDE
2	ABCDE
3	BCD
4	AD
5	B
6	AC
7	ABD
8	ADE
9	ABCD
10	B
11	ABDE
12	ABCDE
13	BCDE
14	E
15	C
16	ACD
17	CDE
18	ABCDE
19	ABCE
20	BC
21	BE
22	BC
23	ACD

Chapter 2

1	ABD

Chapter 3

1	ABD
2	A
3	BDE

Chapter 4

1	ABCDE
2	ADE
3	C

Chapter 4 (contd)

Question	Answer
4	B
5	C
6	ABCDE
7	ABD
8	ABE
9	BCD
10	ABCE
11	BC
12	BE
13	BD
14	ABCDE
15	ABCE

Chapter 5

1	ABCD
2	ABCDE
3	ABCDE
4	ACD
5	A
6	BE
7	CDE

Chapter 6

1	ABC
2	CDE
3	E

Chapter 7

1	ABCDE
2	ACDE
3	CE
4	AC
5	ABC

Chapter 7 (contd)

Question	Answer
6	E
7	ABD
8	BCD
9	ACD
10	BCE
11	ACDE
12	ABCE
13	ABCDE
14	ABCE
15	BCDE
16	ABE
17	ABCE
18	ACD
19	ABCDE
20	ABCD
21	ADE
22	CDE
23	ABE
24	ABE
25	C
26	BCDE
27	ABCDE
28	BCDE
29	ABCE
30	ABCD
31	CDE
32	CDE
33	ABCDE
34	A
35	ABDE
36	ADE
37	ABCDE
38	ABC
39	ABCDE
40	CDE
41	ABCDE
42	DE
43	BCD
44	DE

Question	Answer
1	BCD
2	CDE
3	BE
4	ABC
5	ABCE
6	ABCDE
7	ABCDE
8	CDE
9	ABCDE
10	ABCDE
11	ABCE
12	CDE
13	BCDE
14	C
15	BDE
16	ABDE
17	ABD
18	BCD
19	ABCE
20	ABD
21	ABCE
22	BCD
23	BCDE
24	ABCDE

Chapter 9

Question	Answer
1	BCDE
2	CE
3	ACD
4	AE
5	AC
6	BDE
7	BCDE
8	ABCD
9	ABCE
10	BCDE
11	ABCDE
12	ACD
13	ABCDE

Chapter 10

Question	Answer
1	ABCDE
2	ADE
3	ABD

Chapter 10 (contd)

Question	Answer
4	ABCDE
5	ABCDE
6	BDE
7	ACD
8	ACDE
9	BCE
10	BCDE
11	ACDE
12	ABCD
13	ABCE
14	ABDE
15	ABCDE
16	ADE
17	CDE
18	AB
19	BDE
20	CE
21	ABE
22	ACE
23	ABCDE
24	BDE
25	AD
26	ABE
27	BCD
28	ABCD

Chapter 11

Question	Answer
1	CE
2	ABE
3	AE
4	ABC
5	ACDE
6	ABCDE
7	AD
8	ABCDE

Chapter 12

Question	Answer
1	AD
2	AE
3	ABD
4	ABC
5	BCDE
6	BDE
7	BDE

Chapter 12 (contd)

Question	Answer
8	ACDE
9	ABD
10	BCDE
11	ACD
12	ABCE
13	ABCE
14	ABCD

Chapter 13

Question	Answer
1	ABCE
2	BDE
3	BCD
4	ABCE
5	CD
6	AC
7	BCDE
8	ACD
9	ACDE
10	BDE
11	ABCE
12	ACDE
13	ABCD
14	ABCDE
15	ABCE
16	ABDE
17	ABDE

Chapter 14

Question	Answer
1	AC
2	ABCD
3	ABCD
4	ABCD
5	CD
6	ABDE
7	CDE
8	ABCDE
9	ABCD
10	BCDE

Chapter 15

Question	Answer
1	ABCDE
2	ABCDE
3	BCE

Chapter 15 (contd)

Question	Answer
4	ABCDE
5	DE
6	ABCDE
7	ABCD
8	BCD
9	ACE
10	BCE
11	ABCE
12	BE

Chapter 16

Question	Answer
1	ABD
2	CDE
3	ABCD
4	BE
5	AC
6	AE
7	B
8	AD
9	ABCDE
10	ABCDE
11	ADE
12	BCD
13	ABCE
14	ABE
15	ABCDE

Chapter 17

Question	Answer
1	ACE
2	ABCDE
3	DE
4	ABCDE
5	ABE
6	ABE
7	ABD
8	CE
9	BCE
10	ABCE
11	BDE
12	BCDE
13	ACDE
14	BCDE

Chapter 17 (contd)

Question	Answer
15	ABCD
16	ABDE
17	ABCDE
18	ABCE
19	C
20	ACDE
21	CDE
22	D
23	ABCDE
24	BCDE
25	ABE
26	BD

Chapter 18

Question	Answer
1	ABCE
2	C
3	BCDE
4	BD
5	CE
6	AE
7	BCE
8	C
9	ABCDE
10	BE
11	ABCE

Chapter 19

Question	Answer
1	ABCDE
2	ABC
3	ACDE
4	CE
5	ABCDE
6	ABCDE
7	BCD
8	ABCDE
9	CDE
10	ABDE
11	ACDE
12	ABDE
13	BD
14	DE
15	BCE

Chapter 19 (contd)

Question	Answer
16	CDE
17	DE
18	BCDE
19	CDE
20	ACDE
21	ABCDE

Chapter 20

Question	Answer
1	BDE
2	ABCDE
3	AE
4	ABDE
5	C
6	BCDE
7	ADE
8	ADE
9	BE
10	BCDE
11	ABDE
12	E
13	ABC
14	ABCE
15	ABCE

Chapter 21

Question	Answer
1	ABE
2	BC
3	BCDE
4	CDE
5	ACD
6	ADE
7	BDE
8	ABCDE
9	CE
10	BCDE
11	ABE
12	ADE
13	BDE
14	CDE
15	ABCE
16	CDE
17	ABCDE

Chapter 21 (contd)

Question	Answer
18	ABCD
19	ABCD
20	ABD
21	BD
22	D
23	ABD
24	ACDE

Chapter 22

Question	Answer
1	AE
2	ABDE
3	BE
4	ABCD
5	ABE
6	AC
7	ABD
8	AC
9	AD
10	ABDE
11	ABCDE
12	CD

Chapter 23

Question	Answer
1	ABE
2	ABCDE
3	ABD
4	C
5	BCDE
6	DE
7	ABCD
8	ADE
9	ABCDE
10	ABCD
11	ABCD

Chapter 24

Question	Answer
1	ACDE
2	BCE
3	ACE
4	E

Chapter 24 (contd)

Question	Answer
5	AB
6	AB
7	ACDE
8	BE
9	ACD
10	AE
11	A
12	CE
13	BCDE
14	ACDE
15	D
16	ACDE
17	ABDE
18	ABCDE
19	DE
20	BCDE
21	ACDE
22	ABD
23	AB
24	AB
25	BCD
26	ABCE
27	CDE
28	CD

Chapter 25

Question	Answer
1	ACE
2	A
3	ABC
4	ABE
5	ABE
6	BCE
7	BDE
8	CD
9	CDE
10	ACDE
11	ABDE
12	AB
13	ABCDE
14	ACDE
15	B
16	ACDE
17	ACE
18	ABDE

Chapter 25 (contd)

Question	Answer
19	ABCD
20	BCDE
21	CDE
22	ABCE

Chapter 26

Question	Answer
1	ABCDE
2	BCDE
3	ABCE

Chapter 27

Question	Answer
1	BCE
2	ABC
3	C
4	E
5	AD
6	BCDE
7	ABDE
8	ABDE
9	ABC
10	ABCE
11	ABDE
12	ABDE
13	CE
14	ABCE
15	BDE
16	ABCD
17	AC
18	ABCDE
19	ABD
20	ABCD
21	ABC
22	AC
23	BDE
24	ABCE
25	BD

Chapter 28

Question	Answer
1	ABCE
2	ACDE
3	BCDE

Chapter 28 (contd)

Question	Answer
4	BE
5	BE
6	ABCE
7	ABCD
8	ABC
9	ABCDE
10	BDE
11	BCE
12	D
13	ABCDE
14	ABD
15	ABCD
16	ABC
17	AC

Chapter 29

Question	Answer
1	ABDE
2	ABE
3	ABCDE
4	ABCD
5	DE
6	ABCE
7	ACDE
8	ABDE
9	ABE
10	CDE
11	DE
12	ABDE
13	ABCDE
14	ACDE
15	BDE

Chapter 30

Question	Answer
1	DE
2	ABDE
3	BD
4	BCDE
5	CDE
6	ACD
7	BCE
8	AC
9	ABCD

Chapter 31

Question	Answer
1	ABCD
2	ABCDE
3	ACE
4	ABCDE
5	CDE
6	AB
7	ACDE
8	ABCDE
9	BCDE
10	ABCDE
11	ABCD
12	ABCD
13	ABC
14	ABC

Chapter 32

Question	Answer
1	AE
2	ABCDE
3	BD
4	ABCE
5	DE
6	ACD
7	ABCE
8	AD
9	ABCDE

Chapter 33

Question	Answer
1	BCDE
2	ABDE
3	BE
4	ABDE
5	ABCD
6	ABCE
7	ABCE
8	ABD

Chapter 34

Question	Answer
1	BD
2	ABDE
3	BC
4	ABCE
5	CD

Chapter 35

Question	Answer
1	BDE
2	AC
3	B
4	A
5	BC
6	BCDE
7	CE
8	BDE
9	ABC
10	ABCDE
11	BDE
12	AD
13	ABE
14	ABCD
15	ACDE
16	ABCDE
17	CE
18	B
19	ABCDE
20	ABC
21	ACDE
22	ACDE
23	ABCDE
24	ABDE
25	ACDE

Chapter 36

Question	Answer
1	ABCE
2	ACDE
3	CD
4	ABCE
5	ABCDE
6	ABC
7	B
8	BCE
9	BD
10	ABCDE
11	ABCDE
12	BCE
13	ABCE
14	ABCD

Chapter 37

Question	Answer
1	ABCDE
2	ADE
3	ABCD
4	ABCE
5	ACE
6	ADE
7	AC
8	CDE
9	ABC

Chapter 38

Question	Answer
1	ABD
2	ABCD
3	ABCE
4	AE

Chapter 38 (contd)

Question	Answer
5	BCD
6	BDE
7	ACD
8	ABD
9	BC
10	ABCD
11	A
12	ABD
13	ABCD
14	ABDE
15	CE
16	AE
17	BCDE
18	ABCDE
19	ADE
20	ADE

Chapter 39

Question	Answer
1	ABCDE
2	ABCDE
3	ABD
4	ABCD
5	BDE
6	CD
7	ABCD
8	DE
9	ABCD
10	ACDE
11	BCD